POST **PREGNANCY**
SHAPE UP

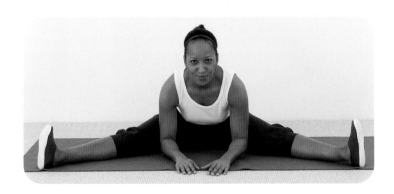

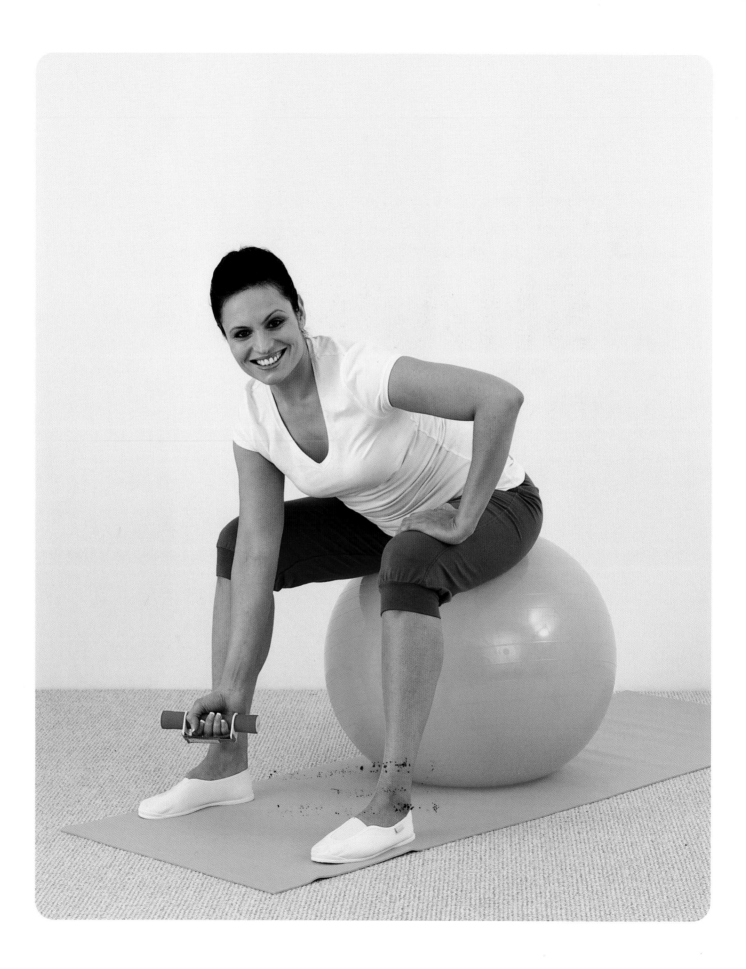

POST **PREGNANCY** SHAPE UP

regain your pre-pregnancy figure
through 10 key exercises

Chrissie Gallagher-Mundy

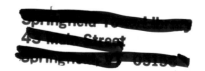

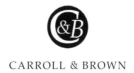

CARROLL & BROWN

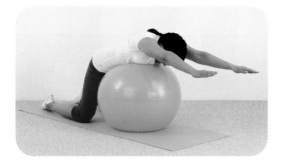

First published in 2013 in the United States by

Carroll & Brown Ltd
20 Lonsdale Road
London NW6 6RD

Library of Congress Cataloging-in-Publication Data

Gallagher-Mundy, Chrissie.
  Post pregnancy shape up : regain your pre-pregnancy figure through 10 key exercises / Chrissie Gallagher-Mundy.
      p. cm.
  Includes index.
  ISBN 978-1-909066-04-5 (pbk. : alk. paper)
  1. Postnatal care--Popular works. 2. Postnatal exercise--Popular works. 3. Abdominal exercises--Popular works. 4. Women--Health and hygiene--Popular works. 5. Physical fitness for women--Popular works. I. Title.

  RG801.G35 2013
  618.6--dc23

                    2012025684

ISBN 978 1 909066 04 5

10987654321

Printed in China

Note: No information provided in this book should be construed as a personal diagnosis or treatment. Always consult with your own physician(s) as regards your own and your child's care.

From me to you 6

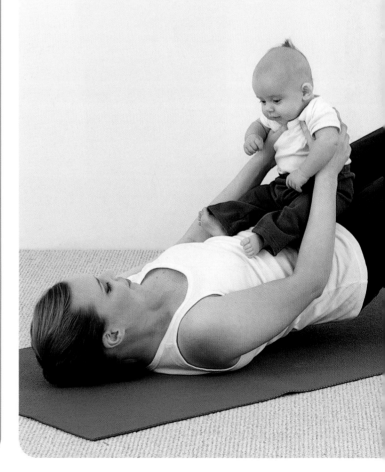

CONTENTS

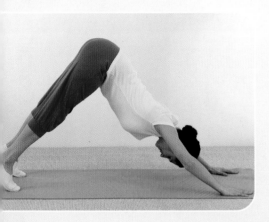

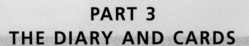

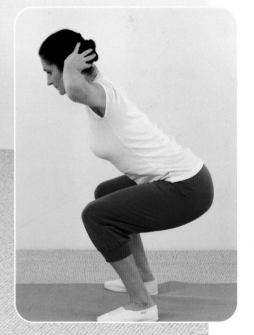

FROM ME TO YOU

Having a baby is an amazing experience. It's one of those fantastical yet natural processes that changes you forever! Once you become a mother, nothing looks or feels quite the same; you experience new emotions, thoughts and ways of looking at things. With all the excitement of these new feelings and caring for your beautiful new baby, it can be hard to concentrate on yourself and remember that your body needs nurturing, too. Your body has just been through nine months of changes and that can take some recovering from. One of the things new moms (and experienced ones too) eventually become concerned about is getting their old body shape back. Often moms worry that their stomach won't flatten out or that they will be left with unsightly fat amassed during pregnancy. Please don't worry! Gaining body fat and the stretching of the stomach area (the abdominal muscles) are all part of the natural process of the body adapting to growing a baby.

This book is designed to take some pressure off you and help you plan a way to fit in some time for yourself and also work (without stress) toward making your body strong and fit again. Your body has already undergone many changes, a (possibly traumatic) birthing process and may now be busy making milk for your newborn. You are also probably tired from lack of sleep and the new demands on your attention so time is at a premium.

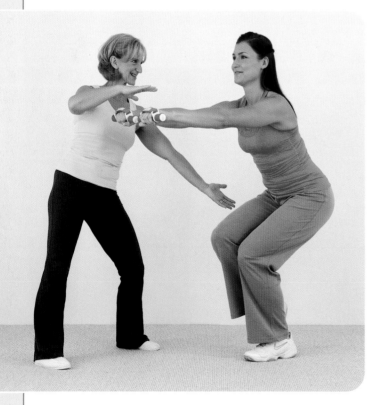

The program contained in this book is simple but effective. You need that because you won't have time to learn complicated routines or master intricate moves—what you will need, though, is a program that progresses over the weeks as you do. The beauty of this program is that you only need to master 10 moves. That's right! In the early stages you are going to learn 10 core moves that will be the basis of your workout throughout the entire 40-week program. Once you have learned the core moves, you will be able to perform them more and more effectively and then challenge yourself even further as they change slightly over the course of the weeks.

The program consists of an evolving workout of 40 weeks' duration. Why 40 weeks? Well that's about how long it took to grow your baby and that's about how long it will take to get your body back to normal again. (Some women, particularly those in their 20s, will regain their previous shape more quickly but even then they need to allow for the fact that it takes time for the body—both internally and externally—to return to normal.)

As the months progress, you will notice that certain exercises will change in their execution to make them more challenging. In the weeks that either an exercise or the complete program stays the same, you should concentrate on increasing the number of repetitions that you attempt. In this way, your program will remain challenging and interesting while being easy to remember and simple to follow.

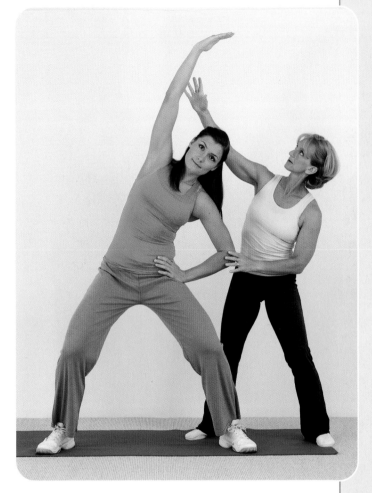

The exercises can be done in any room of the house with a towel, rug, or mat beneath you, or in a gym (if you can get there) and you need very little equipment. Wear clothing that is loose enough to stretch in easily but doesn't hamper movement; place your baby nearby to watch and encourage you.

As you gain strength, regain co-ordination and overcome some of that no-sleep tiredness, you will enjoy this workout that still challenges your muscles to strengthen and shape while ensuring that you stay safe and supple.

Good luck!

Chrissie Gallagher-Mundy

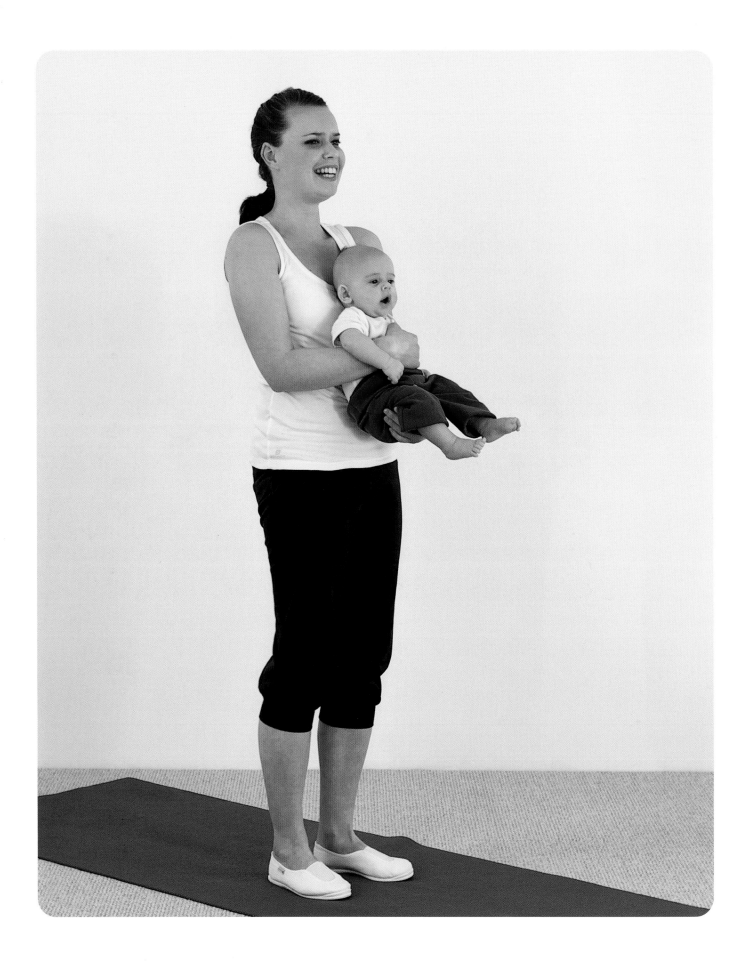

PART

1

Getting Back into Shape

YOUR CHANGING BODY

When you became pregnant, your body had to modify to grow a new human being so all kinds of changes took place. Body systems evolved, changed or enlarged, and hormones and blood flow and composition were affected. Once your baby was delivered, further changes occurred to start the process of returning everything to normal. These processes not only had an impact on internal structures but the way you held and balanced your body during and after pregnancy.

As your growing baby pushed out in front—the abdominals became greatly extended with the central rectus abdominis muscle stretching to around 12–20 inches at full term—you would have noticed a change in your center of gravity. Many women find that as their front is pulled forward, they tend to lean backward to rebalance, and this can cause back discomfort and pain. Once a baby is delivered, this change in the center of gravity needs addressing and work on the abdominals can help to alter alignment of the spine and relieve back pain.

The hormone relaxin (produced by the placenta) also had a profound effect on your body's structure. Designed to increase the flexibility of the pubic symphysis (the small joint at the front of the pelvis) and the ligaments at the sacro-iliac and sacrococcygeal joints (lower back and tail bone) so your baby was able to slide out (in theory!) during delivery, this hormone also affects the rest of the body's ligaments, tendons, and cartilage. All your joints became much more flexible but also less stable. While relaxin will drain away as you progress through the postpartum months, it can remain in the body for five months or more if you are breastfeeding, so you need to take care with any exercise program and make sure that the exercises work you appropriately but don't over-stress vulnerable joints. You need to be particularly careful that you don't over-stretch when you are doing a 'cool down' after exercising as this is when damage can occur; relaxin allows excess stretching that could damage tendons.

Coping with pain

Having a baby is such a body-changing experience that you may be left with a few minor aches and pains afterward. Just because you've had your six-week postpartum check-up, doesn't mean that all your niggles will have gone away. You may have pain from breastfeeding or a cesarean scar or any number of other aches and pains about which you should talk to your doctor to make sure there is no underlying infection or other complication that could affect you or your baby. There are some pains, however, you may need to manage.

Hip pain

Sometimes after a long labor, particularly if your legs were in stirrups, you may have on-going hip pain. Try to move around as much as possible in the early days back at home as this will help your body to return to normal.

Performing the Figure of 8 Scribe (see page 33) can help loosen the hip joints. If the pain is persistent, a warm shower or some massage from your partner in and around the area might bring relief. Some women find a rice sock (see box opposite) can ease odd aches and pains.

Back pain

Back pain is common after pregnancy, particularly around the sacro-iliac joints; this is where the sacrum and pelvis join and articulate slightly to allow the birth of a baby. To locate your sacro-iliac joints, stand upright and place your fingers on your hip bones. Run your

---

WHAT IF YOU HAD A CESAREAN?

More than 30% of mothers in the US now have either an elective or emergency cesarean section to allow for the delivery of a healthy baby. Cesareans are major surgical operations and put greater demands on a mom's body and its recovery at a time when she probably won't be getting much sleep! A woman who has had a cesarean will feel more tired and sore than one who had a fast, vaginal birth with no intervention, and will also need to protect her scar.

If you've had a cesarean, the most important thing to do in the first few days and weeks is to rest (this applies whether you actually went into labor or not). You may also need some help positioning your baby comfortably for breastfeeding. A nurse or lactation specialist should be able to offer advice on this. You can find out more about recuperating from the procedure in my book *Cesarean Recovery* where the key advice is to listen to your body and don't overdo things.

Even though you had a cesarean, you still need to do pelvic floor exercises. Due to your increased weight, the softening of your ligaments and tendons, and the weight of the growing uterus during pregnancy, your pelvic floor muscles will have become stretched and weakened. Therefore you still need to look after this area and tone the underlying pelvic muscles (see page 26).

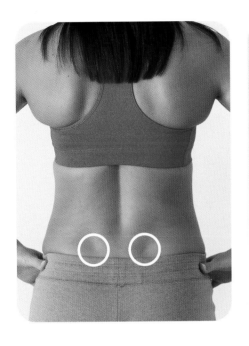

RICE SOCK

A home-made heating pad and ice pack at the ready will mean you are prepared for anything. Take an old, clean, soft, knee-high sock and fill with rice (you could also use corn grain or flax seed) so that the grains can still move around. Tie off the top of the sock to prevent leakage. For a flexible warm pack, place the sock in the microwave for 1–2 minutes (depending on the power of your microwave) and then on or near the area of pain. For a flexible ice pack, place the sock in the freezer for approximately 45 minutes and then place on an area that needs numbing a little.

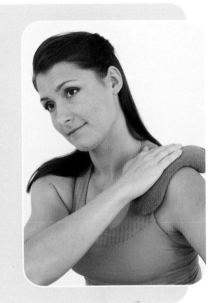

fingers over the top of the bones and trace the line of the pelvis as it goes behind your back, working your fingers down toward your buttocks until you feel two dimples, one either side of your spine (see above). Often, this is an area that remains sore or vulnerable to stress for several months after birth, so be aware of this area and treat it kindly! You can use a rice sock (see box) or heating pad to warm the area. When you stand, stand squarely on two feet rather than throwing your weight onto one hip (easy to do when you're carrying a baby), as this may put too much strain on one side. When you kneel or sit, try to keep the weight between both your hips rather than placing too much weight on one side alone

Perineal pain

After a vaginal birth, you may experience some pain in the area between the vagina and anus. Moreover, this area may be swollen if forceps or a vacuum extractor was used or tender from a tear or episiotomy. Try to take the pressure off this area by lying down when it feels painful. You also can apply a cold pack or take warm baths. This pain should recede over several weeks but if it doesn't, you need to seek medical advice.

Recovering your posture & alignment

The changes your body has undergone during pregnancy can leave you with a "baggy" stomach and out-of-control abdominal muscles.

You have four abdominal muscles that are important for supporting your whole core, allowing movement of this area and shaping and flattening your mid-section.

Your rectus abdominis muscles run vertically down your front—from ribcage to pelvis—and affect flexion of your spine; these are the muscles that have been most stretched during pregnancy (see also rectus diastasis on page 19).

Your internal and external oblique muscles wrap around the waist and cause lateral flexion and rotation of the spine, while your transverse muscle is a deep muscle that runs horizontally across the abdomen, providing deep support to your body's core.

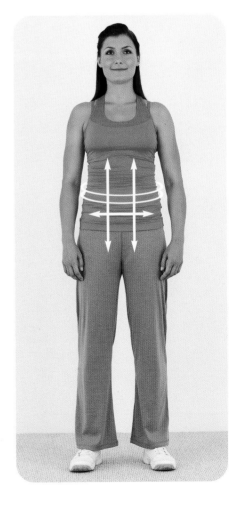

Regain abdominal control

The first thing you need to do is to reconnect your mind with your body, that is, your over-stretched abdominal muscles and your brain. Try the following techniques to help retrain the brain-to-muscle pathway that has been weakened due to pregnancy.

• Lie on the floor with your knees bent and your feet flat on the floor. Place your hands gently across your abdomen and try to contract the muscles away from your hands. Squeeze the muscles in toward your backbone, hold momentarily and then release (see pictures, below).

• Stand upright with your feet hip width apart and hands on your hips. Now suck in your abdominals but also think about flattening them as wide as you can across your hips. Try to feel as though you are widening your hip bones out to the side. Rest and repeat.

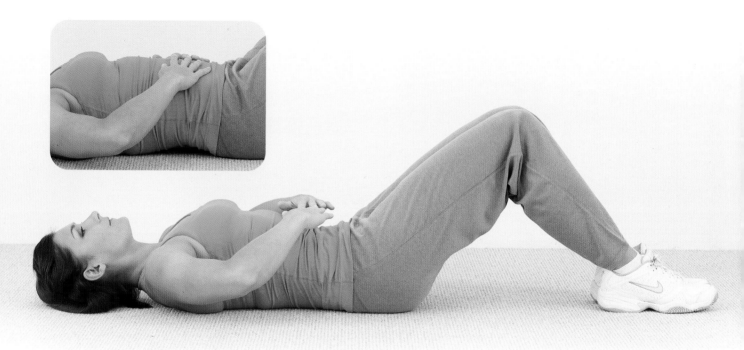

WORKING WITH A PARTNER

If you still have nagging aches and pains, particularly in the back and shoulders, some time after the birth, chances are that there is something wrong with the way you are standing or sitting. If you have decided that you will do some or all of your exercising at a gym, get advice from one of the trainers there. It may be that the smallest adjustment in how you go about your daily routine could make a huge difference. Alternatively, ask a friend or your partner to watch how you stand and move to see if he or she can spot a potential problem.

In addition to having someone else looking out for less-than-perfect posture or technique, working out with a friend can be mutually beneficial and rewarding: you can keep each other going!

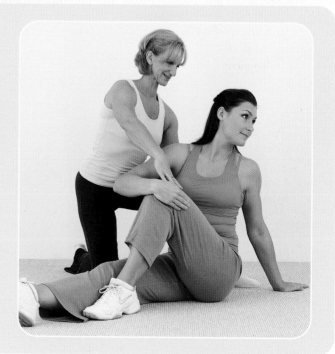

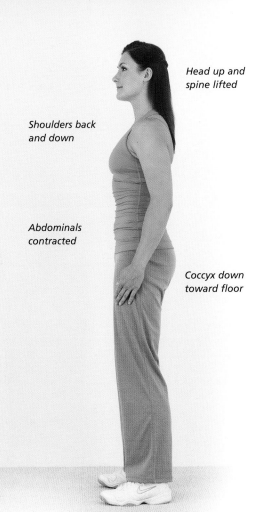

Head up and spine lifted

Shoulders back and down

Abdominals contracted

Coccyx down toward floor

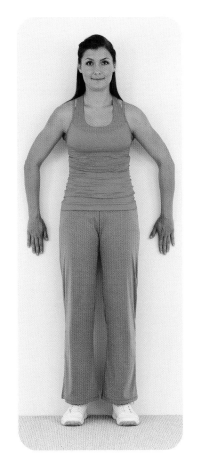

If you find the abdominal muscles that run horizontally, you can use them to keep your core supported. Gently contracting these muscles will keep your whole lower body toned and supported and also protect your lower back.

- Stand upright with your hands on your hips and fingers resting on your stomach. Now cough! The muscles you feel contracting as you cough are your transverse muscles. Now try to re-create that tensing of the muscles without coughing: hold in your stomach as you would if someone was about to punch you.

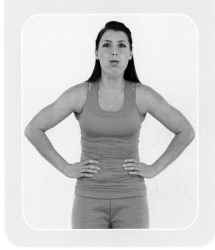

Check your posture and alignment

Twists and strains often happen when bodies move out of alignment and because your ligaments and tendons have been softened, you need to re-check your posture and alignment to avoid any possibility of injury.

- Stand upright against the wall, pressing your shoulder blades back and down behind you and lifting up through the top of your head as if lengthening your whole spine.
- Now press your lower back toward the wall so that you feel your abdominal muscles contracting and flattening. Only press back until you can feel your coccyx pointing toward the floor.
- Take one step away from the wall and try to relax slightly into position.
- Aim to remind yourself of this posture periodically to help the position become instinctive.

- When you bend your legs, in a squat or lunge for example, check that your knees are moving in line with your toes; if your feet are slightly turned out that is the line your knee must follow. This ensures smooth tracking of the joint so that it is not pulling out or in from its natural alignment.

Safe lifting & carrying

Lots of lifting and carrying are involved when you have a new baby and it's a good idea to ensure that you are doing this safely. As you bend, lift, carry, and twist, making sure you are using the right muscles not only will protect vulnerable areas such as your back and hips but you will also tone and firm key muscle groups as you move.

The key areas prone to stress and strain after birth are the lower back, hips, spine, and abdominals. A common injury post birth is when a mother leans over her baby, on the floor or a low surface, and then suddenly stands upright to lift him or her. This can pull the muscles and ligaments around the sacro-iliac joints and cause a lot of pain. To guard against this, it is very important that you learn how to lift and bend in a way that will protect your body from harm.

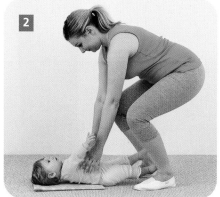

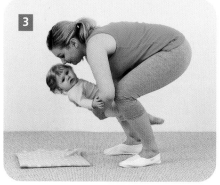

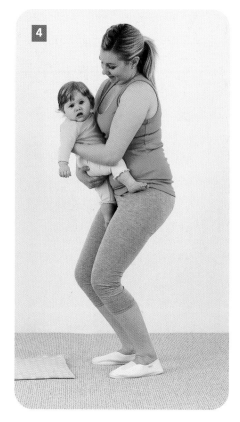

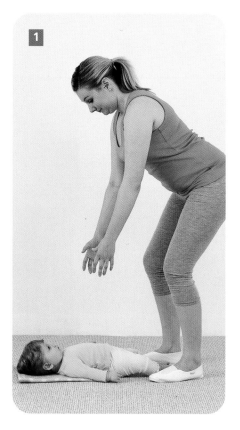

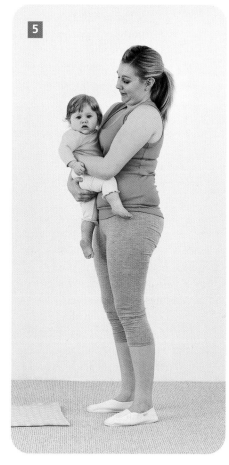

How to lift

It's vital to lift properly and the following sequence is the way to do it. You can rehearse the technique by first practicing picking up a blanket and then with different objects that get progressively heavier. In this way, you will become used to lifting an object with your arms while taking the standing up weight of the lift through your legs. You'll also be strengthening all the major muscles in your legs and buttocks. Once you have mastered the technique, you're ready to lift your baby. Make sure you use this same technique when you bend over your baby, whether to change her diaper on the floor or to lift her in or out of her crib. It may seem odd to stick your bottom out, but lifting this way will keep your back protected and eliminate the risk of strain.

1   Stand upright with your shoulder blades pulled down, suck in your abdominals slightly, and lift your chest. Keep your feet hip width apart and your weight evenly distributed on both feet.Now bend your knees, stick your bottom out behind you and shift your weight over your heels. As you do this, your back should be in a straight line and you should be using your abdominals to support your core area.

2   Bend your legs further to go as low as you need to. At this point, check that your bottom is still stuck out behind you, your weight is on your heels, and your back is straight.

3   Use your arms to pull your baby (or an object) in close to you. (Although a blanket and other things will be lighter than your baby, you still need to practice using your arm muscles to pull them toward you.)

4   Once you have baby close to your body, start to straighten your legs as you hold her securely to you. All the work of pushing up should be in the legs, not the back. Make sure your abdominal muscles are held in tightly.

5   Continue to hold your baby close—supporting the head and neck of a very young baby—until you are fully upright.

EATING, DRINKING & FEELING GOOD

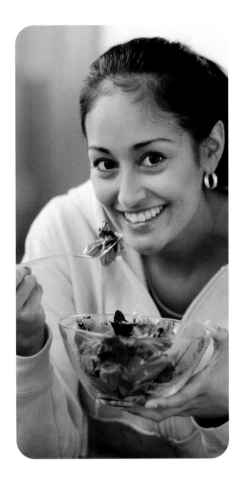

What you eat and drink can help or hinder your body. Eating well becomes even more important when you have been under stress—and being pregnant is one of those times. You want to support your body's recovery in every possible way, and may also need to support your body to produce breast milk.

The eatwell plate helps to set out the basic principles of good eating.

- Choose up to 60% of your foods from the green and yellow sections of the plate. Bread, rice, and other starchy foods contain complex carbohydrates for sustained energy and simple carbohydrates for instant energy. Fruit and vegetables will provide much-needed vitamins and minerals to keep your body functioning well.
- Aim for 5–7 portions from the green section of the plate—and to eat across the rainbow, from red, orange, and yellow through to blue, green, and purple. Eating differently colored produce ensures a variety of different vitamins and minerals (and fiber) are available to your body.
- You also need to choose about 10–15% of your foods from the pink, or protein, section of the plate. Protein is important for growth, balance, and repair but overeating protein is not helpful so stick to the recommended 40–70 g per day— about 1–2 portions. Limit your oily fish servings to two per week.
- Ensure you eat from the blue dairy section of the plate (unless you are lactose intolerant) and choose a range of different products such as milk, yogurt, cheese, and cream. Aim for 2–3 portions per day.
- The small purple section of the plate contains those foods which are high in fat and sugar. Eat the foods in this

section only occasionally—as a treat when you have made sure all your nutritional needs have been covered. Keeping these foods as a low percentage of your diet will ensure that you are not eating too many empty calories and aid weight control.

Fluids

It's also important to have adequate fluids (though caffeinated beverage don't count). Stay hydrated by being aware of your thirst and sipping regularly; don't delay once you notice you are thirsty. Keep a glass of water handy, particularly when you are breastfeeding, but don't feel that you have to drink glasses and glasses constantly; you can over-drink too. Be guided by your body.

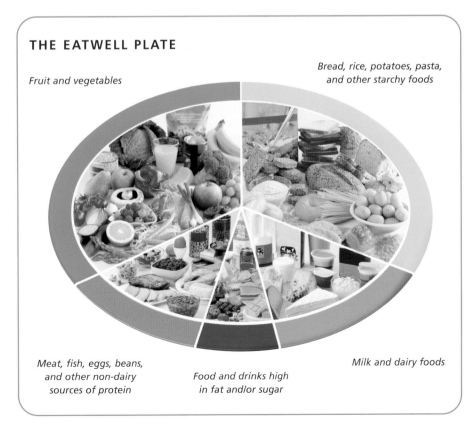

THE EATWELL PLATE

Fruit and vegetables

Bread, rice, potatoes, pasta, and other starchy foods

Meat, fish, eggs, beans, and other non-dairy sources of protein

Food and drinks high in fat and/or sugar

Milk and dairy foods

Looking and feeling better

Getting up and about after you've had your baby will make you feel better almost immediately, but there are plenty of other, simple things you can do to boost your morale from the earliest days back at home.

Work on your posture

Make a point of walking upright and lifted, with your shoulder blades pulled back and down. It is easy, particularly if your breasts are large or milk laden, to hunch over and wander around a little slumped. Try and resist this urge by feeling your head pressing up toward the ceiling, your spine lengthening out, and your chest area "widening". This routine stance will help to strengthen your core, which will turn help to prevent back ache caused by slouching.

Additionally, follow the advice about posture and safe lifting and carrying set out on page 13.

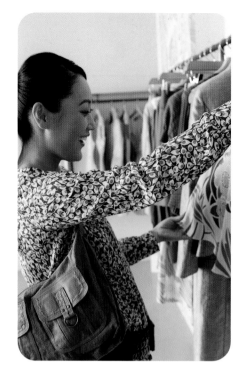

Sort out your wardrobe

If you are feeling that nothing fits then treat yourself to some comfortable casual clothing. There is a lot of stylish leisure wear on the market that allows freedom of movement and is soft and supple on your skin. You want to feel comfortable with loose-fitting garments that can be washed regularly. This kind of casual wear is also ideal for exercising; you can layer it up when it's cold and shrug it off once you are nicely warmed up.

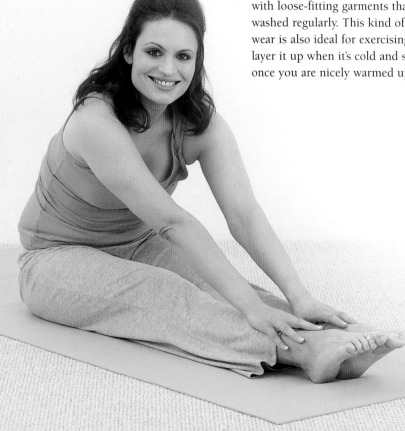

Build up your confidence

If you have a special occasion coming up for which you want to look your best, you may want to check out some of the "shape wear" currently on the market. These undergarments are designed to smooth and pull in rogue bits of flesh so you appear trimmer. There are all kinds of garments that smooth out stomach bumps, cinch in waists, and help thighs appear thinner. These garments aren't an excuse to forget exercise and posture work but they can boost your confidence and self-esteem for a big night out.

Plan for "me time"

One of the most important things for new (or second- or third-time) moms to do is to have some personal time. This means finding space in the day where you do the things you enjoy. Often, early days with a baby are all about the gorgeous new arrival, and it can be hard to grab some private time when you have a steady stream of visitors and haven't had time yet to get into any sort of routine at all. Yet spending time on yourself can be an important part of maintaining a positive mental state and good energy levels. Why not treat yourself to a pedicure or manicure? Your feet have supported a lot of weight over nine months and you may not have seen them in a while! Show them some attention. A hand massage and manicure can be very relaxing and can make you feel miles better if you've been feeling life is all diaper changing and feeding.

Make time for your partner

Ask your partner if he can give you a simple back massage to help boost your circulation and relax your muscles. This can bring you together for a few special moments. Take other time out with your partner when you can just be together so that you don't feel as though you're giving all your time to the baby but are having "couple time" as well as "family time".

EASY FIRST EXERCISES

You may want to wait until your doctor gives you the go-ahead at your post-partum check (usually at around six weeks) before getting heavily into exercise but early on, some gentle exercises may help you to get back in touch with your body and feel in control. When your baby is sleeping or otherwise occupied, do some gentle moving around to get your body going again; this will make you feel more normal and can help relieve lingering aches and pains.

You may feel stiff from time to time if you sit for long periods feeding your baby, so some gentle stretching and mobility work can warm your body up and keep it moving smoothly. By doing a small amount every other day (or whenever you feel up to it), you will start to re-accustom your body to exercise and re-acquaint yourself with your abdominals. You can start to experiment, in the first few weeks with pulling in on your abdominals and trying to re-learn the mind-muscle pathway that previously allowed you to have control over these muscles. If you feel you never had control over your abs, don't panic! This program will help you to locate, feel, and strengthen them.

Stomach toners

While you are feeding your baby, you can tone your abdominals. As your baby suckles, gently contract your abdominal muscles and pull them in as far as you can. Hold for 5 seconds and then relax. Do this 4 or 5 times each time you feed your baby. If you are breastfeeding, your body releases oxytocin that helps shrink the uterus back into your pelvis so contracting your abs while this happens will help further. If you are formula feeding, contracting the stomach muscles will still help flatten your stomach. If you do a set each time you feed your baby you will have done at least 25 stomach pull-ins each day.

Lying on your front

Your stomach and back may feel out of shape and sore so try an experimental lie down to find your body's sensitive areas.

1 Come down onto your hands and knees then stretch out your legs. Slowly walk your hands out and gently lower the front of your body to the floor.

2 Take a moment to register the feeling. If your breasts are enlarged, they may not be comfortable and your midriff may feel sore If you can, put your hands underneath your shoulders and gently press back up to flex your spine and stretch your abdominals.

All fours

Remaining on your hands and knees, press down on your hands as you suck in your stomach and arch your back up toward the ceiling, pressing upward as high as you can. Hold for 5 seconds and then release your back down and this time press your stomach toward the floor as you arch downward, stretching the

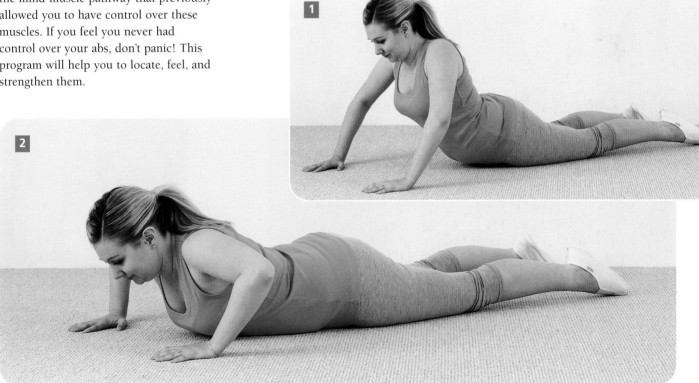

stomach muscle in a different way. Repeat 2–3 times to limber your spine.

Knee rolls

Lie on your back and contract your abdominal muscles. Now, with control, slowly press your knees together and swing them over to one side. If it is comfortable, rest your knees on the floor and feel the gentle twist in your back and the sides of your abdominals. Then lift your knees and swing them over to the other side and feel the stretch across your back and sides on that side. Repeat 4–5 times.

Marching

Hold your baby in your arms and do a little marching on the spot! Put some music on, if you like, and really lift up your knees as high as you can. Work through your feet—toes to heels—and get all your lower body joints warmed up. This is great preparation for your full workout and will get your breathing going, too.

Pelvic floor

Don't forget to do your pelvic floor exercises (see page 26). Again, if you do these every time you feed your baby, you will perform quite a few sets in a day.

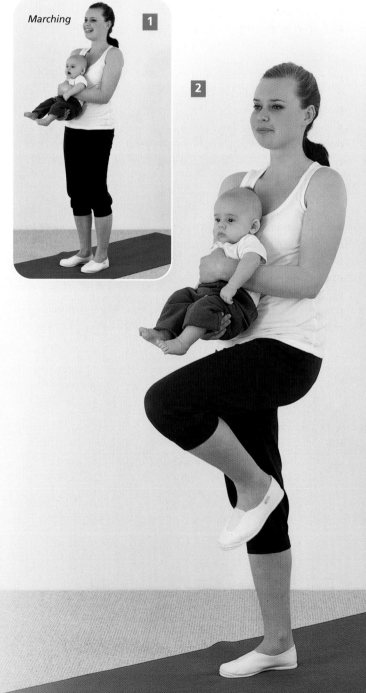
Marching 1

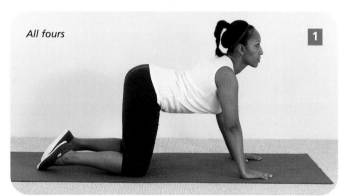
All fours 1

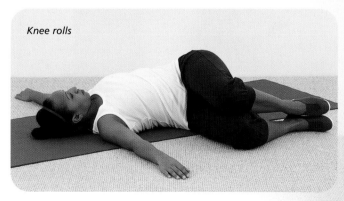
2

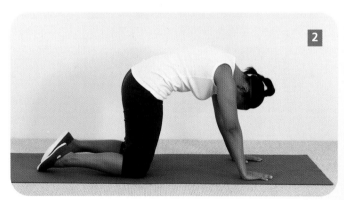
Knee rolls

BEFORE YOU BEGIN

There are many issues you may face after having a baby, including sore muscles or a lack of sleep, but try to stay positive. It's important to understand that despite the adverts on TV and photographs of celebrity moms in the media, most new (and experienced) moms can't do everything perfectly in the first few months. Don't be hard on yourself if you haven't started exercising yet or are unable to wear your pre-pregnancy clothes—it takes time to get back into shape. Bear in mind it took a whole nine months for you to make a baby and may take as long again for you to feel truly back to normal. As you have learned, the body undergoes significant changes during pregnancy, and some of these can take a while to reverse. For example, due to the action of relaxin, the hormone that softens connective tissue, your ribcage may widen slightly leading to a larger waist size than previously. You may also be one of the many women who find that their shoe size has increased; this is due to the relaxing of ligaments and the pressure of your increased weight bearing downward. Be patient and your body will realign in time.

Deciding the exact time to start on the exercise program in this book (or any other exercise regimen) is really up to you. First of all, you want to have visited your doctor for your postpartum check. This should take place at around six weeks. (If you have had a cesarean, the check will probably be about two weeks later, around 8 weeks). The doctor will check your uterus and your blood pressure but you may want to check out your own stomach (see below).

As long as you feel relatively calm and able (even if tired), and any incisions or tears have healed, there is no reason why you cannot start to exercise. Exercising sensibly should not affect your production of breast milk nor should it add adrenalin to it. Start at a time of day when you normally have most energy and when your baby is sleeping or happy to be left in his crib or seat for a while.

Rectus diastasis check

There is one area that needs attention before you start to exercise. A personal trainer can assess this for you but you also can do the check yourself.

When you are pregnant, the rectus abdominis muscles that lie vertically from ribcage to pelvis become stretched and lengthen over the bulk of the growing baby. In some women, these muscles—instead of stretching—pull apart from the linea alba (the central connective tissue that connects the two strips of rectus muscle), leaving a thinning membrane or gap at the center of the abdomen. This is known as rectus diastasis; it is not a serious condition, but it does mean that the core is less well supported.

Performing the check

1 Lie on your back with your legs bent and feet flat on the floor. Press three fingers—held horizontally—into the flesh just beneath your belly button.
2 Lift your head and shoulders just off the floor. As your abdominals contract, you should be able to feel if there is a gap in the muscles. If the muscles are close together, you will feel them repelling your fingers but if you feel a softness under your fingers, suspect that there is maybe a one- or two-finger gap.

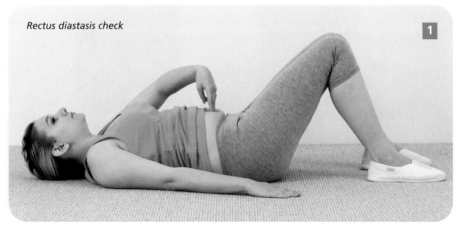

Rectus diastasis check

1

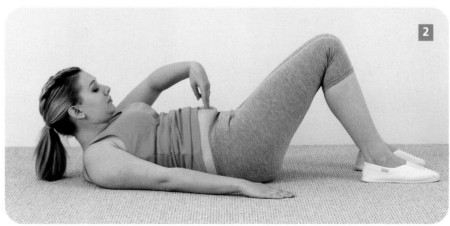

2

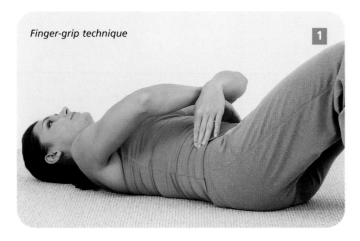

Finger-grip technique **1**

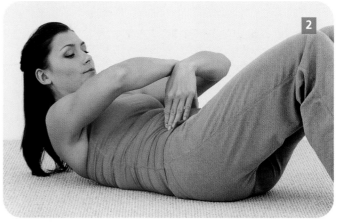

2

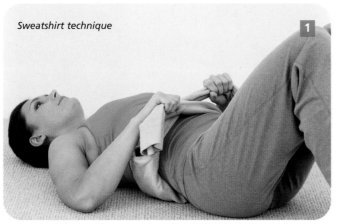

Sweatshirt technique **1**

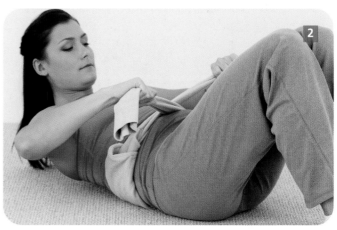

2

Exercising if you have a gap

Having a gap is a perfectly normal state; most gaps are self-correcting and the muscles normally come back together naturally over the first few days after giving birth. Some gaps, however, will remain for longer and if you have one when you begin to exercise—particularly the abdominals—you need to take care of this area during your workout. Two techniques are shown above to prevent you from widening the gap and making it worse while your body works to repair it. Even if you are left with a small gap, your transverse muscles, which are underneath, will keep your core protected and strong. Some of the exercises in the program (for example, the plank series) will strengthen these muscles.

If you are starting the program in this book (or any other abdominal exercises), you can perform the curl exercises (see pages 45–56) but you must place your fingers either side of your belly button and, as you contract the abdominals, use your fingers to pull the muscles together a little (see left, above).

You can also wrap a sweatshirt around your waist and use the arms crossed over to pull the abdominal muscles together as you exercise (see right, above).

A space to exercise

The workout in this book is designed to be done virtually anywhere; you don't need a huge space or a special home gym. You do, however, need an environment that is "friendly" and workable, one where you have enough space to lie flat on the floor with your arms stretched out above your head. When you've found a space, test it out.

You can exercise in your bedroom, kitchen, hallway, and even the bathroom as long as it is safe. Make sure that the room is clear of obstacles that may get in the way as you move your arms and legs around. There should be no hanging or protruding objects that could cause an injury. If you are exercising in the kitchen, don't do so if you are cooking anything on the stove. Also ensure that the room is well ventilated so that you can get some oxygen-rich air into your lungs as you up your pace. Start working in a warm room, if at all possible, as this will help warm your body and not put you off getting started. If the room is carpeted, that is a perfect surface for the floor work; if not, use a mat or a folded towel to lie on.

Think also about where your baby will sit to watch you. Even at a very young age. babies love to watch their moms so if you can arrange things so that you are always able to keep your baby in sight, then you will have a better chance of an uninterrupted workout while providing some entertainment.

CHOOSING A SPORTS BRA

Although you don't have to worry about other items of sportswear, it is important to have a supportive bra while exercising. This is particularly important if you are breastfeeding. When choosing a sports bras, there are a number of things you need to consider, including support and comfort.

Determining the right size

You're almost certainly not the same size you were previously but as this is the most important criterion for a proper-fitting bra, you'll need to make sure you know the correct size to buy.

To find your bra size, use a tape measure and measure around your ribcage directly below your breasts.
To find your cup size, put on a lightweight bra then measure around the fullest part of your breasts. The difference between this figure and your bra size determines cup size. If your breasts are of unequal size, fit to the larger breast. You can always bulk out the less-filled cup with a breast pad.

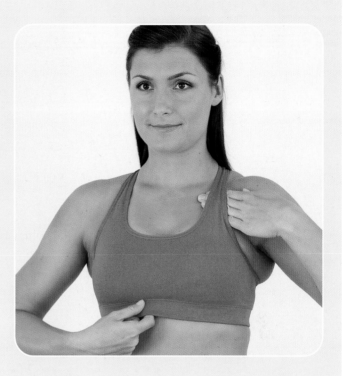

Getting the best fit

Your sports bra will be the same size as your standard bra, but it needs to be much more close fitting. You should just about be able to get a finger under the supportive lower cuff of the bra, which should be tight without cutting into your skin. The stretch will actually increase as the bra is used, so go tighter if in doubt. Sports bras depend on their fabric to compress you slightly, allowing you to move, jump, and run without your breasts bouncing and, for the exercises in this book, a simple compression bra is all you need. If you plan on running, then you should look for a more supportive bra with separate cups in addition to a stretchable, cropped compression design for hold and comfort.

Style

Simple sports bras are generally of the racer-back type, though it is possible to find ones more like standard bras. Racer backs offer more support over the back, so they feel tighter and really secure. The fabric for sports bras is usually synthetic—polyester mesh or lycra are the most common as these are more capable of wicking away sweat than cotton. Mesh provides breathability and ventilation, which is ideal for circulating air.

Comfort

Sports bras lack underwiring and often are put on like a crop top—that is, they may not have hooks and eyes— so it's important that you are comfortable putting it on and taking it off. Make sure that any straps or fastenings do not dig into your skin—particularly under your arms— and that the stitching, seams, and any under-bust support bands are soft and unlikely to cause rubbing and painful friction against your skin. Always try on the bra before you buy and do a few practice jumps in the changing cubicle to see how the bra fits and feels!

YOUR CUP SIZE

0 in (0 cm) = A	
1 in (3 cm) = B	
2 in (5 cm) = C	
3 in (8 cm) = D	
4 in (10 cm) = DD	
5 in (13 cm) = E	
6 in (15 cm) = F	
7 in (18 cm) = G	
8 in (20 cm) = H	

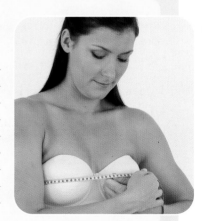

Suitable clothing

Don't stress about what you wear to work out. If you have workout gear then make use of it; if nothing fits or it is old, don't worry. Just find some pants and a T-shirt that will not hamper your movement. You want to wear something in which you can move freely and preferably dress in layers so that as you warm up, you can take off outer layers to stay comfortable.

Your pace

Be aware of how you feel during and after your first workouts. This is all part of keeping your program challenging but

WEIGHTS

Many women are put off lifting heavy weights because they fear becoming big or bulky, even though weight training is one of the most beneficial kinds of exercise for both women and men. The vast majority of women don't have enough testosterone to build bulky muscles, so this should not be a worry. What you should worry about is maintaining muscle tone, which gives you shape and uses up calories. As you age, your muscle mass declines significantly unless you stimulate its maintenance by performing weighted exercises. Muscles will provide strength and shape as you age and, more importantly, improve your ability to carry out functional tasks. Having had a baby you are extra lucky because your baby can act as a "dumbbell," constantly getting heavier. Try some of the weighted exercises you know from this book or from your gym holding your baby securely in both hands. Move him or her around; you will really notice the weight after a few minutes!

also safe. During the workout sessions, you should feel that you are working quite hard and that muscles are getting used. If you have worked muscles hard that haven't been used for a while, you may experience some stiffness afterward. You may even experience DOMS. This is delayed onset of muscle soreness that comes on over a period of two to three days and can really make you ache. This soreness will recede after a few days, but if it's really bad, you could take a mild analgesic to ease the process. If you do the program as instructed, however, and build up gradually, you should be able to avoid any real painful stiffness.

If you do feel particularly exhausted after a workout session, you may want to scale the program back a little; only do half the amount of repetitions, for example, or only do half the exercises. Your body will tell you what feels right so try and tune into that information and this will keep you working out without being put off by exhaustion.

Eating and drinking

Try to eat a couple of hours before you begin exercising, if at all possible. This reduces the risk of indigestion and will ensure you have energy to get the most out of your exercises. Stop frequently throughout your session to take sips of water and, at the end of a session, take a further half glass full. This will keep you hydrated and feeling well.

You may even need to pause your workout to feed your baby. Don't worry about doing this, as it will keep the baby happy so you can then carry on!

Breathing techniques

Before you begin your workout, make sure you are making the most of your breath. The main muscles used in breathing are the diaphragm, which is a large flat domed muscle that lies at the bottom of the lungs, and the intercostal muscles (external and internal), which lift and lower the ribcage to draw air into and out of the lungs. The intercostal muscles run in different directions

between the ribs and help move the ribcage up and down so air can be breathed in and out. The more you exercise regularly, the more you tone these muscles (like every other muscle) so they become more efficient at allowing oxygen into and out of the body.

There is a theory that we don't utilize enough of our lung space when we breathe and often shallow breathe when we should be breathing deeply. Try lying on the floor and taking some breaths that you observe. You should see your stomach as well as your lungs swell slightly. If you don't, then try to breathe more deeply and allow your stomach area—as well as your lungs—to become involved.

Pursed lip breathing

You can also try this type of breathing, which is considered to allow more oxygen into the body. It's a good technique to use if you are feeling breathless as it helps to control your breathing a little. Breathe in and count: "one birthday, two birthday" then, when you breathe out, purse your lips and release the air through this narrowed gap counting: "one birthday, two birthday, three birthday" or until all the air is released.

Finding the time

As a new mom, you will always be pushed for time but there may be periods in the day when you have some minutes to yourself or when you feel you have more energy. These are the times to attempt some exercise. Although exercise routines require time and energy, they give back twofold. Fitting in just a little movement will give you extra reserves of energy and allow you to better cope with stressful situations.

If you feel that fitting in exercise is too difficult, try to approach it differently by breaking up your exercise into short bouts. Thinking about squeezing in an hour of exercise may seem daunting yet if you split your sessions into 10- or 15-minute segments, they may seem more manageable.

EQUIPMENT NEEDS

The exercises in this book make use of a few pieces of equipment, which are readily available in gyms if you're doing your program outside the home. If working at home, you can buy them all online or from sports and fitness shops. All, except for the ball, can be improvised.

- **A mat** is useful for comfort and protects your bony spine. If you don't own a mat, use a rug or several towels.
- **Steps** are available with or without risers that allow you to work at different heights. If you invest in one with a riser, you can adjust the height of the step to increase the intensity of your workout as you progress. If you don't want to invest in a manufactured step, you could try using any small, stable, raised surface such as a well-supported plank.
- **A barbell** is a weighted stick to which you can attach further disc-shaped weights. If you don't want to invest in one, try using a broom or mop.
- **A dumbbell, barbell, or free weight** can be replaced by bottles of water, bottles filled with sand or any heavy household object (like a can of food) that you can hold easily in one hand. See also box on weights on page 22.
- **A Swiss or exercise ball** is inflatable (and deflatable for storage) and usually come with a special pump. If yours doesn't, you can either buy a separate pump, use a mattress pump, or take it to a gas station and inflate it there using their air machine.
  Only inflate your ball to the recommended diameter, which is printed on the ball. Most

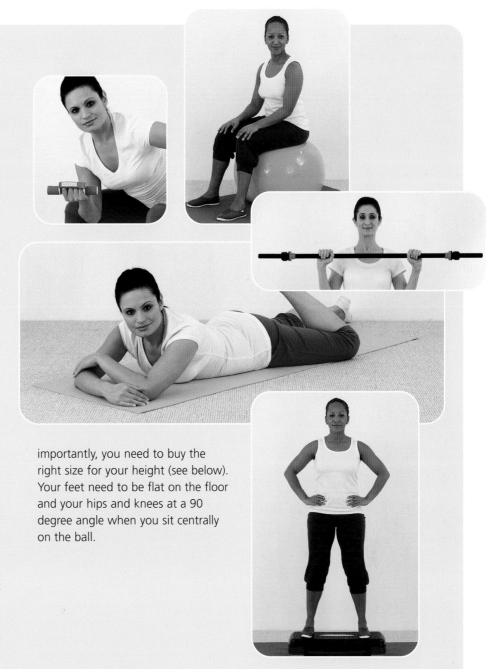

importantly, you need to buy the right size for your height (see below). Your feet need to be flat on the floor and your hips and knees at a 90 degree angle when you sit centrally on the ball.

BALL SIZE GUIDE

Your height	Ball diameter	
4 ft 11 in to 5 ft 4 in (1.5 m to 1.64 m)	21 in (55 cm)	
5 ft 5 in to 5 ft 11 in (1.64 m to 1.82 m)	25 in (65 cm)	
6 ft+ (1.82 m+)	29 in (75 cm)	

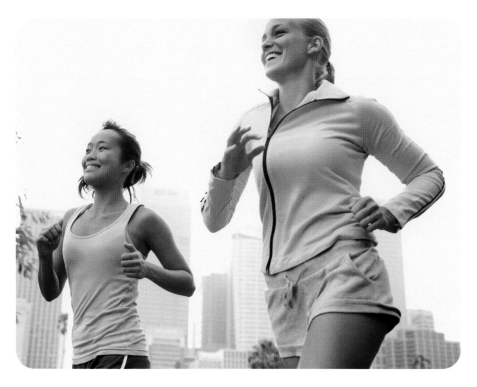

BORG SCALE

How hard are you working?

0	Nothing at all
1	Very light
2	Fairly light
3	Moderate
4	Somewhat hard
5	Hard
6	
7	Very hard
8	
9	
10	Very, very hard

Recommended guidelines are 150 minutes of exercise every week (five 30-minute sessions), including moderate-intensity aerobic exercise and at least two sessions of muscle-strengthening activities. The 30 minutes, however, can be broken down into 10-minute or longer sessions of moderate or vigorous effort and still make a difference to your health.

Alternative ways to exercise

As well as following the workout programs in this book you can try to fit in some additional exercise while you are getting other things done.

Walking

This is one of the best and easiest ways to build your cardiovascular fitness. You can walk carrying your baby in a sling and can build a routine that develops over a number of weeks. Each time you walk (at the mall, for a local errand), you can use this method to walk at a speed that challenges your cardiovascular system and builds your stamina and endurance.

1   Start by walking at a pace that feels comfortable and easily "do-able." Walk upright, swinging your arms and breathing regularly through your

mouth. Walk heel-toe and try to roll through the foot, pushing forward with each step. Now assess how hard you feel you are working: on a scale of 1 to 10, if 1 = nothing at all and 10 = very, very hard (see Borg scale, above). How hard do you really feel you are working? Make a mental note of this and move on to stage 2.

2   Once you have established an "easy" stride, start to up the pace a little. Step faster; the faster you swing your arms the faster your legs will go. Try to get yourself up to a rating of 7 (on your 1–10 scale). To do this, you will have to really push the pace, move your arms and breathe deeply.

3   Once you are familiar with what these intensities feel like, you can start to experiment with different ones when you walk. Set yourself a time—say 30 minutes—and within that time frame, do a warm-up pace of say 2 on the scale then segue into a moderate pace of 4–5 and then, when you are ready to push yourself a little, aim for a 7 or even an 8 for several minutes. Always do a "warm down"—a couple of minutes where you gradually slow the pace—rather than stopping suddenly.

Getting started with jogging

If you have enjoyed fast walking you may be ready to start jogging. Jogging entails more impact on the joints (and probably more discomfort for the breasts and stomach), but there is no evidence that it is bad for joints. Once you have built up your stamina by walking briskly and building up your intensity by working your way up the Borg scale you can try some jogging.

You can take your baby with you in a stroller and push this and jog at the same time. There are specific models you can buy, which are aerodynamically designed for jogging, but any well-made stroller should suffice and you'll probably find your baby will love the motion and probably drop off to sleep as you jog.

If you have never jogged before, below you will find a very simple way to get started. One word of caution: wear a sports bra with plenty of support especially if your breasts are heavy with milk. If you do get strains or stresses, rest and restart when you feel more comfortable.

- Grab yourself a stop watch and set it for 5 minutes. Leave your house and jog down the road at a slow pace that you feel you can maintain.

- As you begin to get breathless, slow down if you need to but keep jogging (don't stop or walk) and give your body time to adjust. Your body is working its way through its energy systems and you have to give it chance for the aerobic energy system to kick in.

- When you have jogged (however slowly) for 5 minutes, turn around and jog straight back. In 10 minutes you will have done a great little workout and be at home again.

- Stay with 5 minutes each way (or less if you need to) for three sessions and then add a minute or so. In this way, you can build your distance up slowly but manageably, and within a few weeks you could be running miles.

Working out with a stroller

If you want to do some different kinds of exercises you've got an excellent tool to use. You can use your baby's stroller to add resistance to your walks or as an aid to other exercises.

Use the handle like a ballet barre. Holding onto it for balance, try the following:

- Lift one leg and swing it backward and forward to warm up your groin muscles. Repeat by turning around and swinging your other leg.

- Pick up your outside leg and swing it in a figure-of-8 shape (see page 33).

- Attempt some squat moves from pages 72–74 of the core exercises. Keep your back straight and your

hands on the handle as you bend and straighten your legs. (Always keep your heels down!)

- With both hands on the handle, walk your feet backward until you are bent over and your back is parallel to, and your eyes are facing, the ground. Feel a pleasant stretch around your shoulders, lower back, and the backs of your legs (hamstrings). Contract your abdominals and then walk your feet back in again.

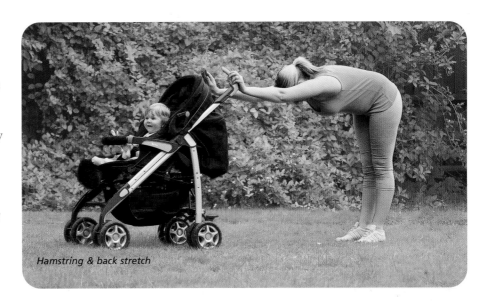

Hamstring & back stretch

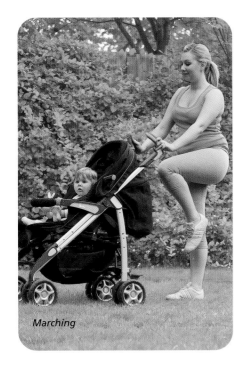

Marching

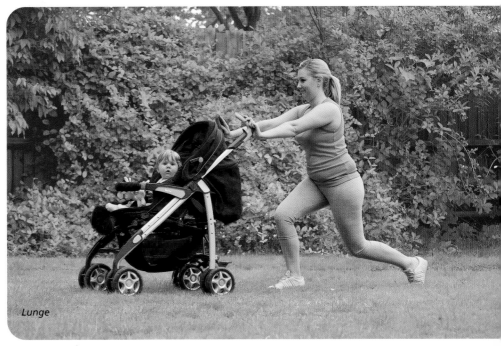

Lunge

Exercising your pelvic floor

Your pelvic floor muscles are a sling of muscles that support your vagina, bowel, and bladder. A double layer of both deep and more superficial muscle runs from the front of your pelvis to the base of your spine and helps to provide stability for the whole of the pelvic girdle. Consequently, they are a vital part of what is regarded in fitness as the "core."

The pelvic floor muscles support the weight of your internal organs and that of your baby when you are pregnant. They are key in keeping you continent, and help with defecation and sexual intercourse. During a normal vaginal delivery, these muscles will be stretched to their utmost to enable your baby to come out. These muscles come under a lot of pressure in pregnancy, too. The good news is, as with all muscles, they respond to exercise so it is as important to have a pelvic floor workout as it is to have a full body workout.

Ideally, you should exercise your pelvic floor throughout pregnancy but if you didn't—don't panic; you can do them now and still tone them. Try these exercises (also known as Kegels) several times a day to ensure your coccygeal and levator ani pelvic floor muscles become strong and flexible again. You can sit, stand, or walk while doing them as no one can see what you're doing. If you haven't done them before, however, you might want to sit or kneel in a position that allows you to feel these muscles more easily.

If possible, you should exercise your main abdominal muscles at the same time. Performing the rectus diastasis check (see page 19), would have put you in touch with these abdominal muscles and using excellent posture when standing, will remind you of your pelvic floor. When you stand, get into the habit of contracting your abdominals slightly, pulling the coccyx down toward the floor, lifting your ribcage up off your waist, and pulling your shoulder blades back and down. If you do so whenever you contract your abdominals, you will

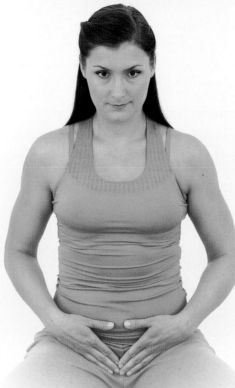

want to pull up on your pelvic floor muscles, as these work in concert with the abdominals, and you will feel "lifted" from underneath as well as at the front.

If you feel tension in your shoulders or tense them when under stress, try to get into the habit of transferring the contraction to your core by pulling in on your abdominal and pelvic floor muscles to support your lower stomach area. You will appear relaxed while working your abs and relaxing your shoulders.

Finally, you have to remember to do your pelvic floor exercises so use a cue to remind you. For example, going to the toilet should prompt you into doing some pelvic floor contractions. Once you have emptied your bladder, you can do a quick 10–20 contractions. If you do so every time you use the toilet, you will chalk up 80–100 repetitions daily—a thorough workout for rhese muscles.

Squeeze and short hold

Start by just pulling up on the muscles underneath the pelvic floor—the ones you use to stop yourself from urinating or during sex—and holding for the count of five. Don't hold your breath or pull in your abdominal muscles; concentrate on just pulling up those pelvic muscles. Release and repeat 8–10 times.

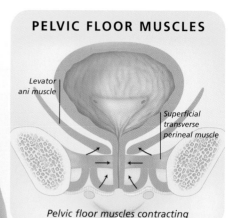

PELVIC FLOOR MUSCLES

Levator ani muscle

Superficial transverse perineal muscle

Pelvic floor muscles contracting

Squeeze and long hold

Try squeezing your pelvic floor muscles and holding for a count of 10–15, then slowly release the muscles for a count of 10. Follow this with quick flick contractions (a contraction that is not held but is just a brief squeeze that's quickly released) for eight repetitions then relax and repeat.

Three-way workout

You actually have separate rings of muscles around the urethra, vagina, and anus. Try squeezing the muscles just around the urethra (and nowhere else), hold, and then release. This is probably easiest while urinating to begin with but try not to interfere with the urine flow too much as it could cause an infection. Now contract the muscles around the vagina and then release, and finally contract those around the anus and then release. Alternate between squeezing the muscles around the different openings to fully work the whole area. Do 10–20 repetitions in total.

Squeeze and change

Try squeezing your pelvic floor muscles (feeling as if you are stopping yourself urinating) and then hold onto that contraction while you change position. Go from sitting to standing or standing to crouching and see if you can keep those muscles contracted throughout. Repeat 8–10 times.

Adding other fitness components

You should now be feeling that you have your get-back-in-shape plans well in hand. You have your full get-fit program in this book as well as advice on walking and jogging, exercising with a stroller, and working on your pelvic floor. What you should aim to do is benefit from all the different components of fitness discussed here.

As well as forming part of the book's program, they can be achieved with other activities as indicated.

Cardiovascular fitness

This involves using your heart and all the vessels that carry blood, oxygen, and nutrients to all your body's cells. If you add the efficiency of your lungs to this equation, then it is termed cardiorespiratory fitness. The kinds of exercise that work this system include walking, running, skipping, dancing, hiking, stepping, jumping, cycling, rowing, treadmill jogging, and cross training, among others.

Another easy way to exercise this system is by rebounding—using a small trampette or mini trampoline on which you bounce up and down. Running, jogging, and jumping movements can be done on this with very minimal impact on the joints. The bouncing is reported to be very beneficial to the system and the uneven surface is good for your balance too! Trampettes are not expensive to buy and can be found in most fitness shops.

Muscular endurance

This is the component of fitness that focuses on making sure your muscles can contract again and again against resistance so that you keep going. Muscular endurance increases when muscles are repeatedly used and stressed, so the more you work them, the more your muscles will be able to endure. Any movements against resistance will work your muscular endurance; this includes body-weight exercises such as push ups and curl ups, and also weighted workouts with light weights and lots of repetitions.

Muscular strength

Also involving your muscles, this component of fitness is about your body's ability to lift heavier objects and your muscles' ability to contract against a heavier resistance. Building strength means you are less likely to pull or strain muscles when you suddenly lift something heavy, and will help you to maintain your shape and posture. Try doing weighted exercises (for example, the ones illustrated in this book) with heavier weights than indicated—heavy enough so that you can only do 8–10 repetitions. Working with your own body weight for resistance, such as with press ups, or with equipment such as weighted wrist or ankle balls or bells will also build strength.

Flexibility

It can be easy to overlook the flexibility component of fitness, but it's important to include some stretches and mobility work as part of your fitness routine. Mobility work (for example, the exercises found in the warm up section of this book, pages 32–33) are good to do at the beginning of a workout because they warm up the joints and get the body going. Stretching, which is all about lengthening the muscles, is great to do at the end of a workout (see pages 82–83), because it returns the muscles to their pre-exercise length. You can also, at a later stage, work on extending your flexibility by staying in the stretches a little longer, thereby further lengthening your muscles.

Motor skills

Additional exercise components consist of balance, co-ordination, power, speed, agility, and reaction time. You can inject these into your workout as you become more competent.

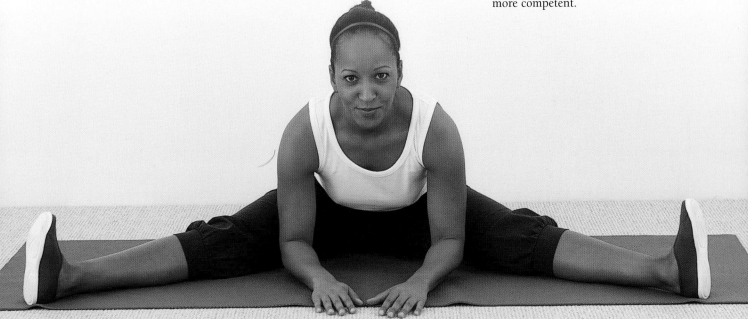

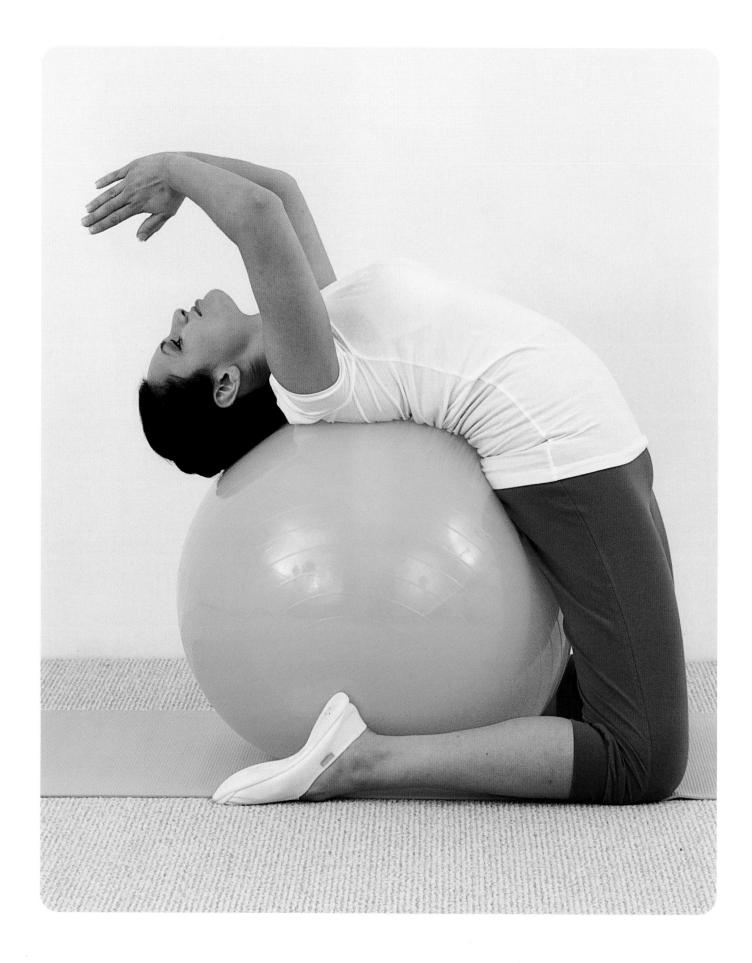

PART

2

The Shape Up Program

YOUR PROGRAM

The great thing about the *Post Pregnancy Shape Up* program is that it is not complicated. Each week, for 40 weeks, you will perform a trio of warm-ups and cool-downs and each of the 10 core exercises—either the basic pose or a variation—as set out on the relevant program card.

The program is designed to be easy to follow, but if you have any question at all about it, you can email me using chrissie@lapf.co.uk.

Good luck with your endeavors and congratulations on your growing, beautiful baby!

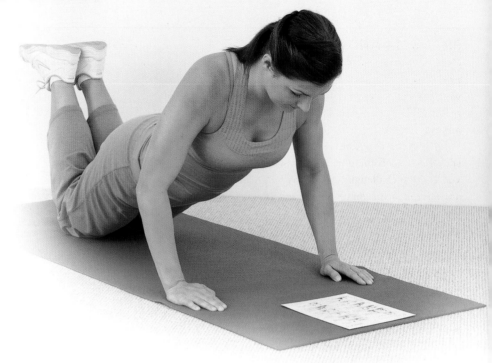

WARMING UP AND COOLING DOWN

Every workout in the program begins with a series of exercises to get your muscles warm and ready for the coming exercises. Similarly, each workout ends with some stretches to cool you down so that you do not stop working abruptly.

WARM-UPS
loosen up the arms, hips, and legs and stretch out the chest area so you can move smoothly and lessen the risk of injury.

COOL DOWNS
target your triceps, hamstrings, and the oblique abdominal muscles at the sides of your waist, to stretch them out and keep them supple.

CORE EXERCISES
The exercises have been designed to give you a full body workout while concentrating on the abdominals. Take your time to learn the steps for each exercise—they are all fully illustrated and described—so that you can be sure you are doing the moves correctly. Make sure you are comfortable with how each one should be performed. Start with the basic poses and, when you reach a changing point, perfect the next variation.

STEP
will exercise your heart and lungs and improve your circulation.

PLANK
builds strength around your core.

CURLS
tighten and strengthen your abdominal area.

HYPEREXTENSION
helps keep your abdominal muscles stretched out and strengthens your back muscles.

ROLL DOWNS
flex and mobilize your spine.

PRESS UPS
can work the chest and arm muscles, abdominals, and buttocks.

THIGH TONERS
do just that—targeting the outer and inner thigh muscles.

SQUATS
strengthen and tone the quadriceps and hamstring muscles of the lower body.

LUNGES
are great body strengtheners, targeting the thigh, gluteal, and calf muscles and challenging your balance.

BODY STRETCH
lengthens muscles, maintains your range of movement, and normalizes blood flow.

PROGRAM AND CARDS

Once you feel ready to begin, you will find your weekly program cards at the back of the book; each card contains two weeks of the program. The cards are peforated and can be removed if you want to take them to another room or the gym and then stored in the back of the book.

As the weeks progress, your program will change—but only slightly—to become more and more testing, which will enable you to keep challenging your body and improve your fitness and overall shape. Some moves will need to be practiced for many weeks while others will alter frequently. Where an exercise doesn't change, you may want to "up your effort" by practicing more repetitions. If at any time you want to remain at a particular week or go back to a previous version of an exercise, then do so until you feel strong enough to progress.

If you possibly can, aim to repeat each week's program 2–3 times in a week, ideally not on consecutive days. This gives you the best chance of getting back into shape in a reasonable time frame. If, however, you can only find time for one workout session a week (especially near the beginning), this will also bring benefits, although more slowly.

YOUR SHAPE UP DIARY

The diary (see pages 84–93) gives you the opportunity of setting and recording your own goals and progress. The program goals are a key part of your post-pregnancy recovery, but your own goals are important, too. Your goals are personal to you and only you know what is most important at any point in the coming weeks and months as you grow into your new role of "mom."

You can also use these pages to note down what's going well in the program and what you are finding challenging. Most women will find some exercises and variations easier than others at different times, so this is your chance to keep your own record. The diary gives space for you to record what you do every day: on workout days, fill in what you actually did, for example "managed 10 reps" or "bit of a struggle but did it all today." You could also put down how you felt—"exhausted!" or "really energized!"

Finally, use these pages to jot down what you did on non-workout days that made you feel good (or not!). For example, "great new smoothie recipe" or "walk in the park," or "actually joined gym today." Many women keep a "pregnancy diary;" this is your chance to keep a "getting back into shape" diary.

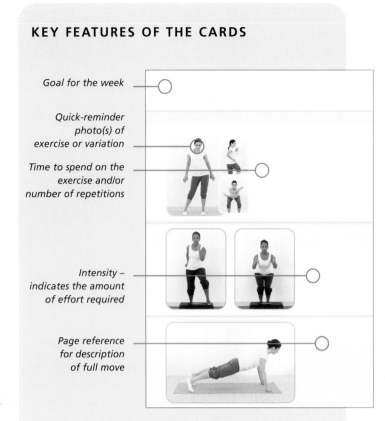

KEY FEATURES OF THE CARDS

Goal for the week

Quick-reminder photo(s) of exercise or variation

Time to spend on the exercise and/or number of repetitions

Intensity – indicates the amount of effort required

Page reference for description of full move

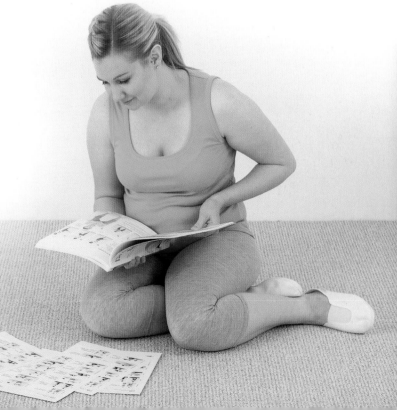

WARM UPS

SHOULDER & HIP CIRCLE

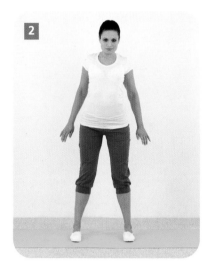

Lift your shoulders up toward your ears as high as you can then push them back, pulling your shoulder blades down in a circular motion.

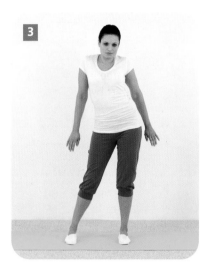

Keep doing this forward and backward circling movement while you start to move your hips.

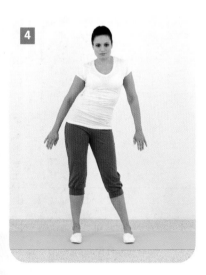

Move your hips in a large wide circle—pushing out as far as you can in each direction.

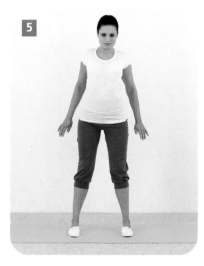

Circle the hips and shoulders together until you can feel the joints warming and becoming easier to move.

Start in a lifted upright position: back straight, shoulder blades pulled down the back, ribs lifted off the waist and abdominals pulled in.

FIGURE OF 8 SCRIBE

1 Stand next to a wall on one leg; place your hand on the wall to help you balance.
2 Move your free leg in a figure of 8 shape. Start by turning inward and swinging your foot across your supporting knee.
3 Then turn outward in a wide arc swinging your foot behind your supporting leg and out around the back to complete the second half of the figure. It may take some practice to make this movement smooth. Repeat using your other leg.

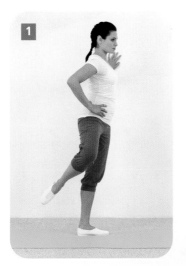 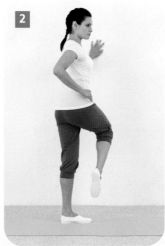 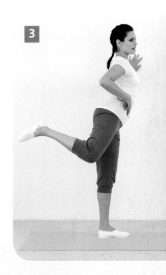

SQUAT & SWING

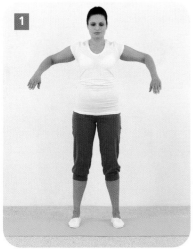 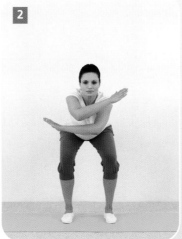

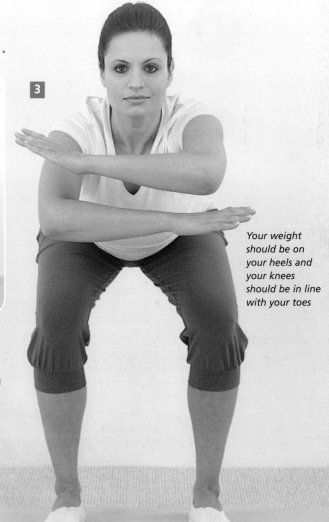

Your weight should be on your heels and your knees should be in line with your toes

1 Stand tall and swing both arms out to the side of your body so that you feel a gentle stretch across your chest.
2 Now bend both legs sticking your backside out far behind you as you squat downward. Swing your arms one way across your chest as you hit the lowest point.
3 Swing your arms out to the other sides as you straighten up. Repeat.
4 Keep the movement smooth and don't swing your arms too vigorously.

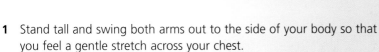

STEP

This cardio booster will get your breathing going and your heart pumping.

Make sure your step is on a non-slip surface and that the surrounding area is free of objects that might get in your way. You can, however, place your baby in front of your step so that you can keep an eye on her/him and s/he can have something interesting to watch while you do your workout!

TIME **3–4 minutes**
INTENSITY **moderate**

Keep your upper body lifted and back of your neck long

BASIC STEP UP

1 Start in a lifted, correct posture position (see page 32).
2 Step up onto the step with your left foot.
3 Follow with your right foot.
4 Then step back down with your left foot and down with your right. Your rhythm is: left, right (both feet on step); left, right (both feet off step). Swing your arms in a natural rhythm (right arm up with left foot; left arm up with right foot) as you build up pace and move faster as you feel more confident.

For variation, try leading with the other foot.

Swing your arms and build up quite a speed!

Try putting on some music to get a good rhythm going

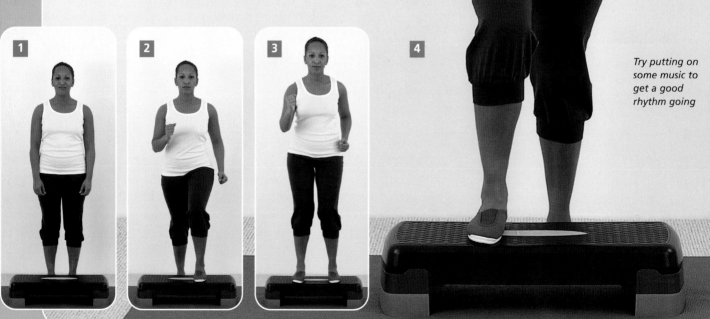

VARIATIONS

WITH KNEE LIFT

This can be done from week 4

1 Step onto the step with your left foot.
2 Lift your right knee up high to meet your left elbow.
3 Put your right foot on the floor followed by your left foot.
4 Turn to the opposite corner of the step. Step up with your right foot.
5 Lift your left knee up high to meet your right elbow. Put your left foot on the floor followed by your right foot.

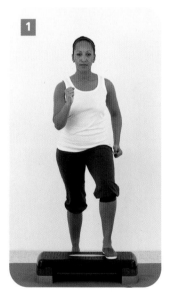

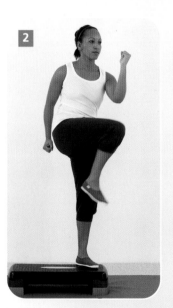

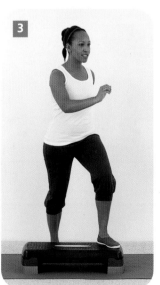

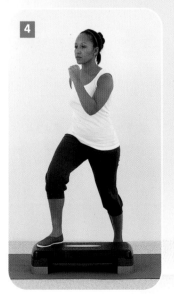

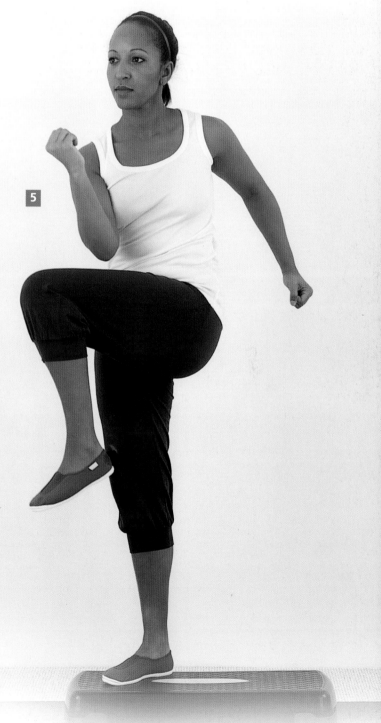

WITH SQUATS

This can be done from week 8

1 Step out wide onto the top of the step with your right foot.

2 Step out wide onto the top of the step with your left foot.
3 Bring your right leg back down to the floor.
4 Then bring your left leg down onto the floor and as both legs come together, squat down and bend both legs for extra work.

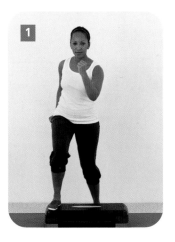
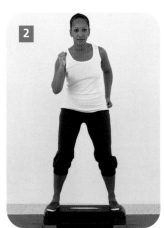
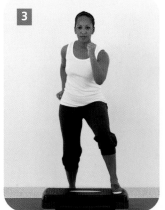
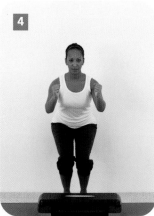

WITH KICK

TIME **2 minutes** INTENSITY **moderate**

This can be done from week 12

1 Step onto the corner of the step with your left leg.
2 Bring your right leg up and kick out toward the corner of the room.
3 Step back down onto the floor with your right leg and then your left.
4 Repeat sequence starting with your right leg on the corner of the step.

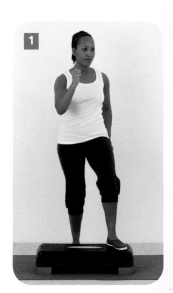
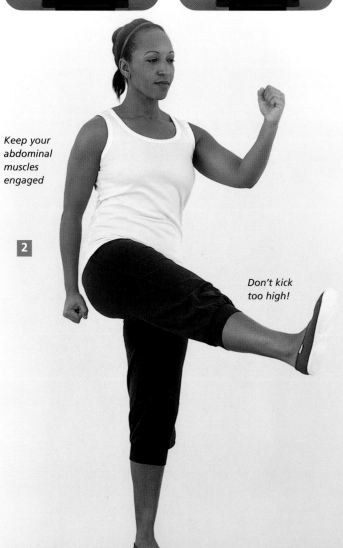

Keep your abdominal muscles engaged

Don't kick too high!

SIDEWAYS

TIME **2 minutes** INTENSITY **moderate**

This can be done from week 15

1 Stand on top of your step facing one end.
2 Step down to the floor with your left foot.

3 Step down to the floor with your right foot.
4 Step back up again with your left foot and repeat the sequence.

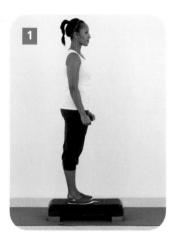
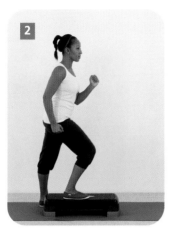
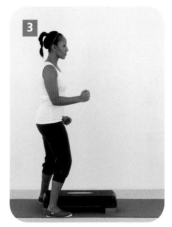
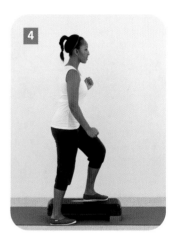

WITH JUMPS

REPS **10** INTENSITY **vigorous**

This can be done from week 22

1 Stand on the top of your step facing one end.
2 Step down to the floor with your right foot.

3 Step down to the floor with your left foot.
4 Bend your knees, swing your arms and jump with both feet back onto the step.

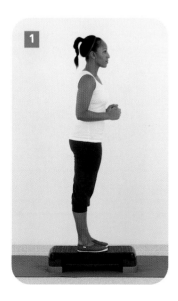
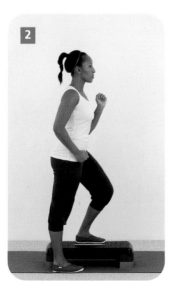
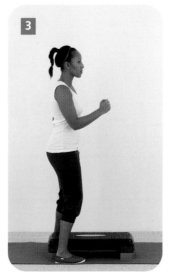
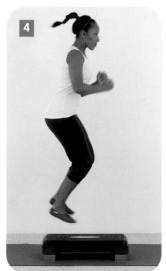

QUICK TIME

This can be done from week 28

1 Stand on top of the step ready to move from side to side of it.
2 Touch your left leg down to the floor on the left side of the step.
3 Briskly bring it back to the top of the step while touching your right leg down to the floor on the right side of the step.
4 Briskly bring your right leg back to the step and touch your left leg down.
5 Continue moving swiftly between left and right legs and on and off the step with a skipping motion.

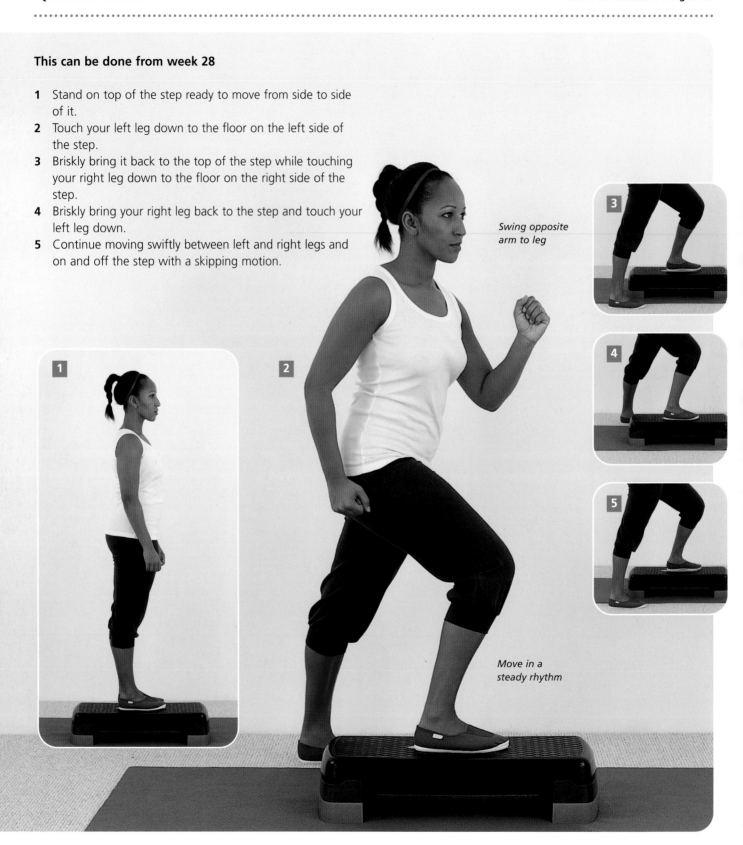

Swing opposite arm to leg

Move in a steady rhythm

PLANK

These exercises are very important for building strength around your middle. This mid section of your body—the abdomen at the front, the sides of your waist and your back—is referred to as your "core." Toning the muscles in this area helps to support your internal organs and spine more effectively, thereby reducing pain. Toning the abdominals flattens out the tummy area helping you to regain your pre-pregnancy shape. The latest thinking is that working on the deeper abdominal muscles that cross the abdominal area will help to draw in and support the front and back of the body. Getting these muscles strong again is particularly important after pregnancy when this area has been stretched and strained after carrying a growing baby for nine months.

TIME **Hold the position for 20 seconds**
INTENSITY **moderate**

BASIC BABY PLANK

In the early days of regaining your strength, you need to start slowly with the plank exercises, so that you don't overstrain your back.

- Get into position by resting on your forearms and your knees. Raise your hips about 2 inches off the floor and tense your abdominal area. Breathe naturally as you hold this position.

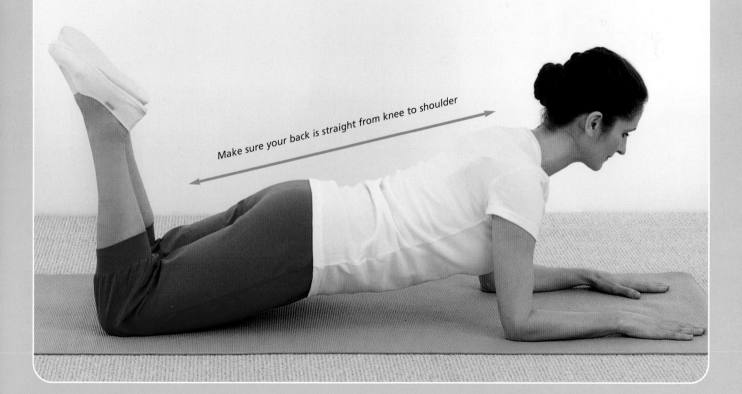

Make sure your back is straight from knee to shoulder

PLANK VARIATIONS

3/4 ON KNUCKLES

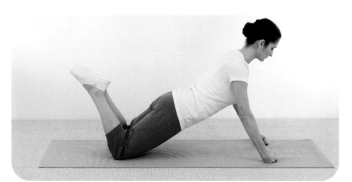

TIME **20 seconds** INTENSITY **moderate**

This can be done from week 2

- Assume the basic baby plank position (see page 39) but make fists of your hands to take your weight onto your knuckles and strengthen your wrists. Tense your abdominals to keep your back straight. If you prefer, you can place your hands flat.

FULL PLANK

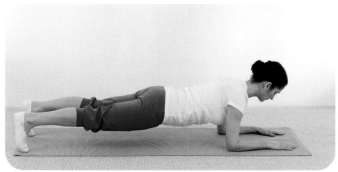

TIME **20 seconds** INTENSITY **moderate**

This can be done from week 4

- Place your forearms flat on the floor and stretch out your legs behind you. Lift your knees off the floor and balance on your toes, taking your weight on your forearms. Tense your abdominals to keep your back straight.

FULL PLANK ON KNUCKLES

TIME **30 seconds** INTENSITY **vigorous**

This can be done from week 8

- Assume the basic baby plank position (see page 39) with your forearms flat on the floor. Make a fist of your hands and place your weight on your fists. Extend one leg and then the other to balance on your toes. Draw in your abdominal area to keep your back straight.

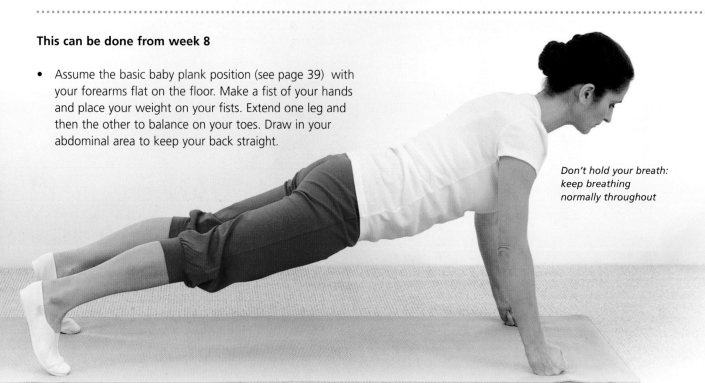

Don't hold your breath: keep breathing normally throughout

FOOT LIFT

TIME **30 seconds (with lifting and lowering of foot)** INTENSITY **vigorous**

This can be done from week 12

1 Assume the full plank position as in week 4 (see opposite page). Transfer your weight onto your right foot and lift your left foot off the floor.
2 Slowly lower your left foot and repeat with your right foot.

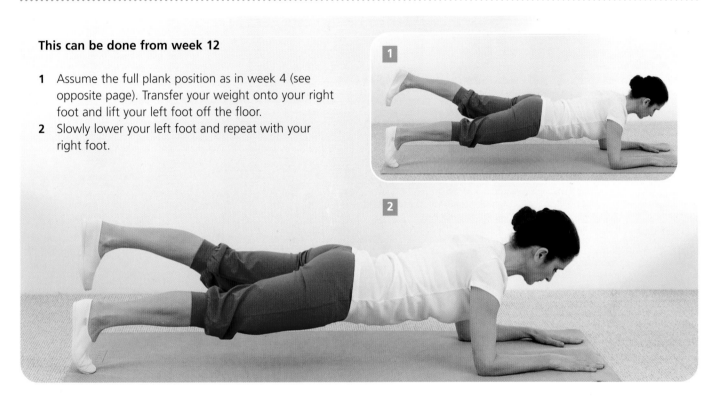

STEP IT

TIME **30 seconds (while moving feet)** INTENSITY **vigorous**

This can be done from week 16

1 Assume the full plank position (see opposite).
2 Walk your left foot out to your left side.

3 Walk your right foot out to your right side.
4 Then walk your left foot back to the middle, followed by your right foot. Repeat this pattern of "out, out, in, in."

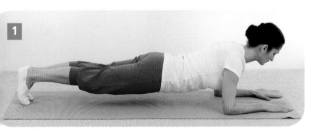

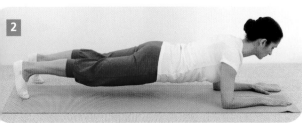

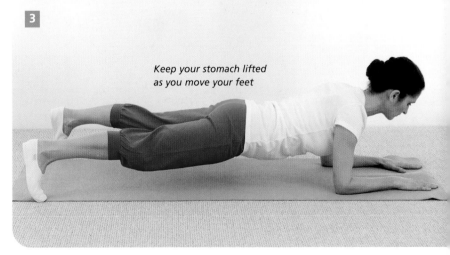

Keep your stomach lifted as you move your feet

STEP UPS

This can be done from week 20

1 Starting with both feet on a step, assume the full plank position (see page 40). Tense your abdominals to hold your back straight.

2 Take your right foot off the step and place it on the floor.
3 Take your left foot off the step onto the floor.
4 Then lift your right foot back onto the step, followed by your left. Repeat this pattern of "down, down, up, up."

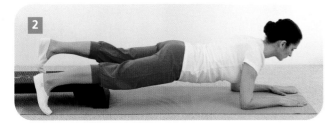

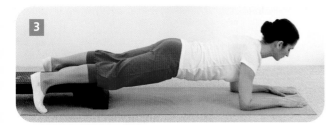

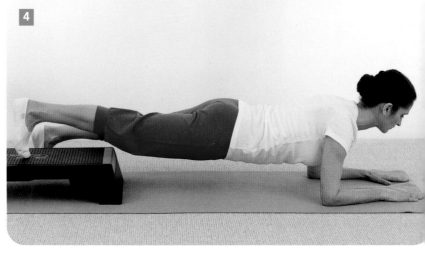

TOUCH LINE

This can be done from week 24

1 Assume the full plank position (see page 40), concentrating on contracting your abdominals to support your mid section.

2 Now gently reach your right arm out to the side and touch your fingertips to the floor.
3 Move this arm back in again and reach your left arm out to the side and touch your fingertips to the floor. Repeat.

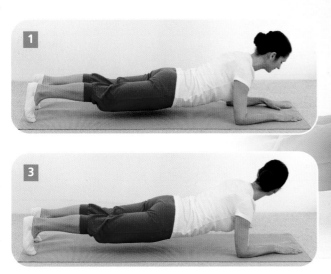

Try not to twist too much but keep your hips facing the floor

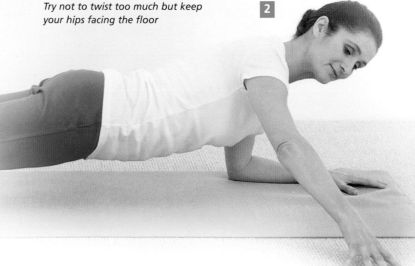

SEMAPHORE

TIME **30 seconds (while moving arms)** INTENSITY **vigorous**

This can be done from week 27

1 Start in full plank position (see page 40).
2 Lift and extend one arm in front of you, keeping it straight out in front.

3 Move your arm out to the side before putting it back on the floor.
4 Repeat the motion with your other arm, all the time keeping your mid-section lifted.

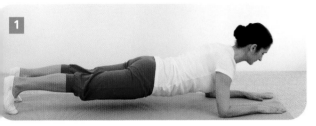

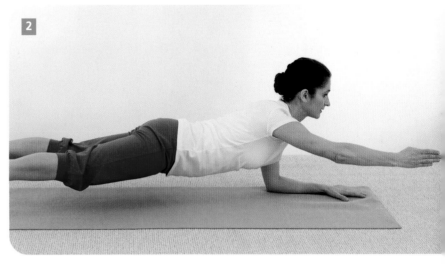

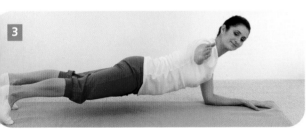

V-LIFTS

REPS **10–15** INTENSITY **vigorous**

This can be done from week 32

1 Start in a raised plank position on flat hands.

2 Now contract your abdominal area sharply so that your hips are lifted high into the air
3 Lower, with control, back into the flat position and repeat.

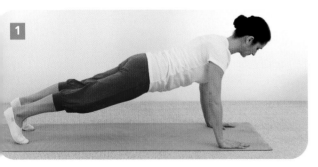

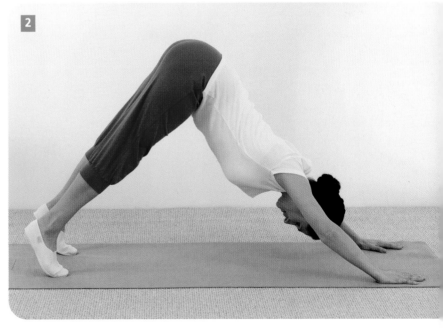

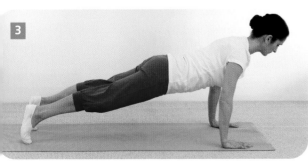

MOUNTAIN CLIMBERS

This can be done from week 36

1 Start in plank position on your flat hands and bring one knee across your body and try to touch it to the opposite elbow. Don't worry if you can't actually touch the elbow.

2 Take your knee back then bring your other knee across to touch the opposite elbow. The mere act of trying will tone and challenge your core muscles!

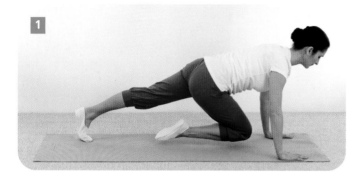

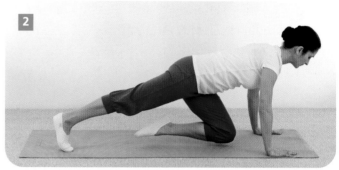

SPIDERMAN

This can be done from week 40

This is a tough exercise so don't worry if you don't get it right away!

1 Start in plank position with arms slightly bent. Bend one leg and lift your knee right up to the side of your body. Imagine you are climbing a high wall (like Spiderman) and you need to get your leg up really high.

2 Now straighten your arms and place your foot back down (return to plank position).

3 Repeat with your other leg.

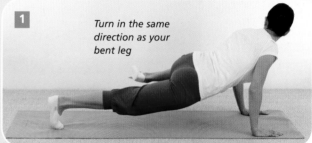

Turn in the same direction as your bent leg

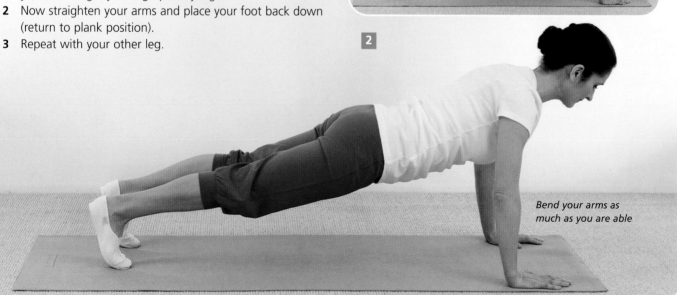

Bend your arms as much as you are able

CURLS

The curls series of exercises will tighten and strengthen your abdominal area. After pregnancy, your abdominal muscles are stretched and stressed so they need some loving care to encourage them back into shape! The main longitudinal muscles that reach from the bottom of your ribs down to your pelvis—the rectus abdominis—are the muscles that become most stretched in pregnancy and can sometimes pull apart (see page 19) but the external obliques, the internal obliques, and the transverse muscles of the abdominal area, also have been stretched so any exercises that encourage the entire group to tighten and pull in are good.

When you begin to do any curl-up exercise, your first goal is to flatten the muscles as you start to engage them. The basic curl and flat curl variation (from week 2) will help you grasp this so that each exercise not only strengthens your abdominal muscles but helps re-educate them back into flatness.

REPS **5**
INTENSITY **moderate**

BASIC CURL

1 Start by lying on your back with feet flat on the floor.
2 Now slowly curl your head and shoulders off the floor as you slide your hands up your thighs.
3 Gently release back down to the floor again.

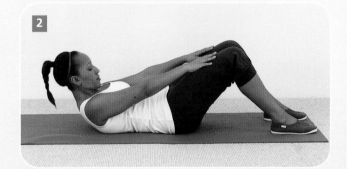

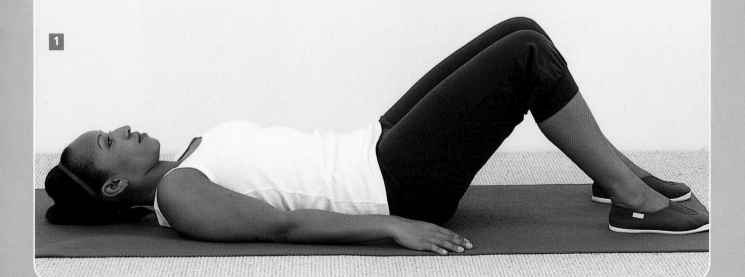

VARIATIONS

FLAT CURL

This can be done from week 2

1 Lie on the floor on your back with knees bent and feet flat on the floor. Place your hands on your abdomen.

2 As you begin to lift your head and shoulders, try to pull in your abdominals at the same time. You should feel those muscles contracting and flattening under your hands.

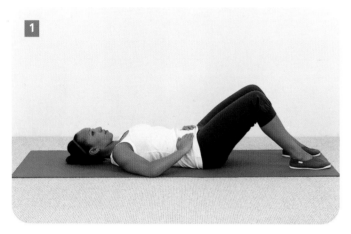

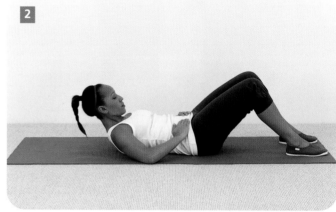

FULL CURL

This can be done from week 6

1 Lying flat on the floor with your feet hip width apart, place your hands behind your head.

2 Lift your head and shoulders off the floor and hold briefly in the lifted position, gazing at the ceiling.
3 Lower your head and shoulders slowly back down and repeat.

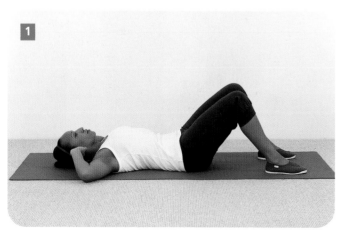

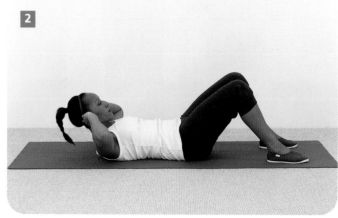

BALL AB CURL

This can be done from week 10

1 Begin by sitting upright on a ball, hands by your bottom, and legs out in front.
2 Walk your feet out and slide your back down the ball until you are lying backward over it. Place your hands by your ears.
3 Now, from this extended position, contract your abdominals to bring you up in a curl.
4 Release back over the ball and repeat.

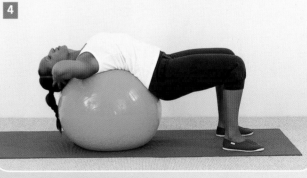

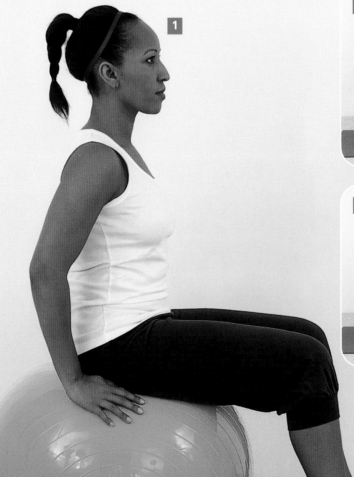

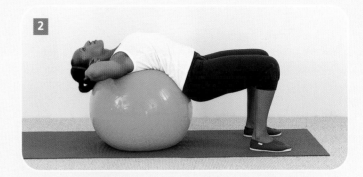

Extra work for fully extended abdominals

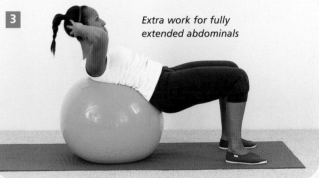

5 To come up off the ball, roll your back over the ball and walk your feet so that the ball rolls back underneath your bottom and you are able to assume an upright sitting position.

KNEE CURL

This can be done from week 14

1 Lie flat on your back with your hands behind your head and legs bent in front.
2 Now, as you curl your head and shoulders off the floor, bring one knee up toward your chest.
3 Lower your knee and upper body to the floor at the same time.
4 Repeat with your other leg.

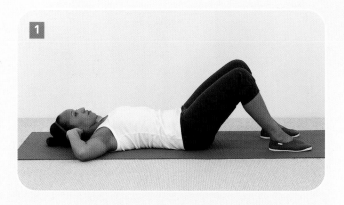

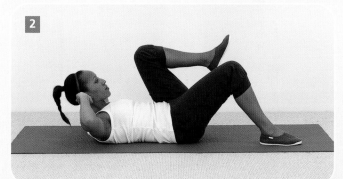

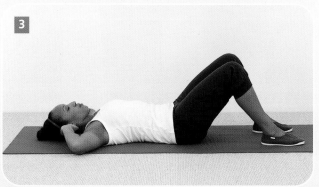

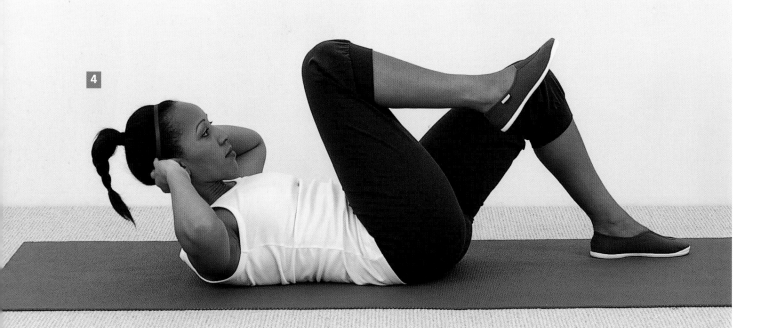

DIAGONAL CURL

REPS **15 on each alternating leg** INTENSITY **moderate**

This can be done from week 18

1 Lie on your back with your hands behind your head and, as you curl your head and shoulders off the floor, lift one knee across your body and try and touch it to the opposite elbow.

2 Release back down then curl your other knee across your body to touch the opposite elbow.

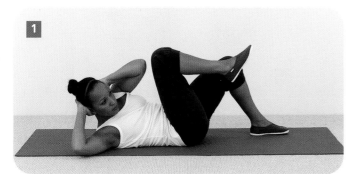

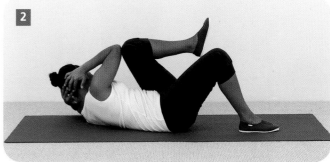

WEIGHT LIFT

REPS **20** INTENSITY **moderate**

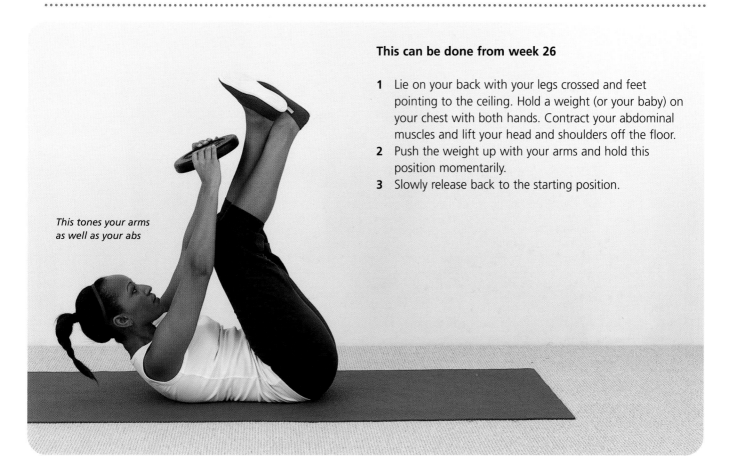

This tones your arms as well as your abs

This can be done from week 26

1 Lie on your back with your legs crossed and feet pointing to the ceiling. Hold a weight (or your baby) on your chest with both hands. Contract your abdominal muscles and lift your head and shoulders off the floor.
2 Push the weight up with your arms and hold this position momentarily.
3 Slowly release back to the starting position.

LOWER AB TIGHTENER

This can be done from week 30

1 Lie on your back with both legs bent at right angles, feet off the floor; you can place your hands across your abdominal area to become more aware of the muscles.
2 Now slowly lower one heel to touch the floor.
3 Then bring the leg back up.
4 Now slowly lower the other heel to touch the floor.

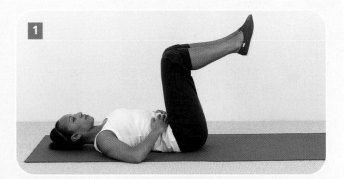

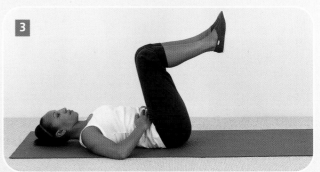

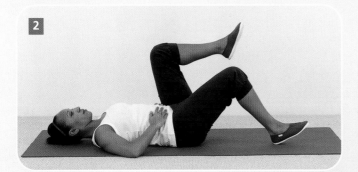

The real work is when you struggle to keep your lower back pressed well into the floor as you lower each leg

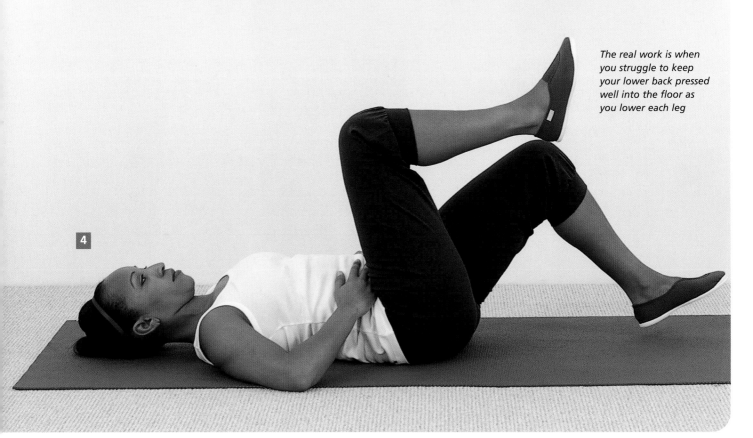

BALL AB BUSTER

REPS **10** INTENSITY **vigorous**

This can be done from week 33

1 Start by standing with the ball in front of you then bend forward over the ball and place your hands on the far side. Roll your body over the ball until only your lower legs are balanced on the surface and the rest of your weight is on your hands.

2 From this extended position, contract your abdominals sharply and bend your knees so that the ball rolls up underneath you.

3 With control, release the ball back away from you until your legs are straight and back in the start position.

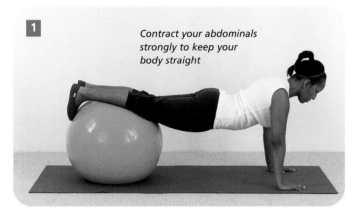

Contract your abdominals strongly to keep your body straight

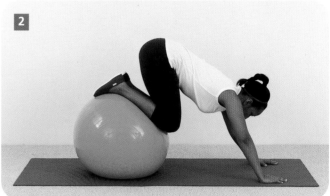

HALF V-SIT

REPS **15 on each leg** INTENSITY **vigorous**

This can be done from week 34

1 Lie on the floor with both arms extended, one leg straight and the other bent.

2 Contract your mid-section strongly and lift up your upper body and your straight leg. Try to reach your foot with your hands.

3 Lower back down, with control, then repeat step 2 with your other leg.

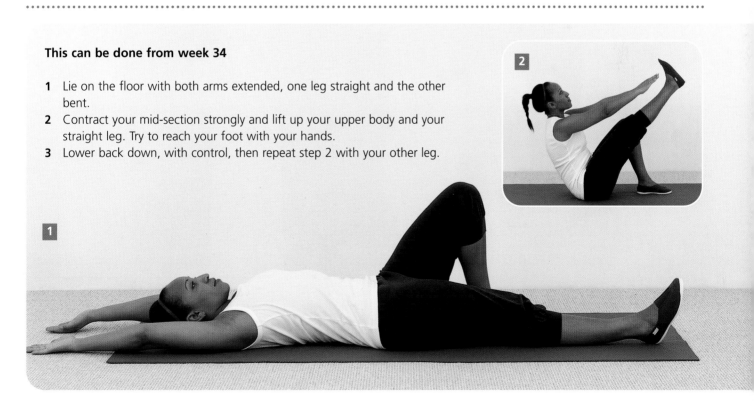

FULL V-SIT

This can be done from week 36

1 Start by sitting up, knees bent, and your feet just touching the floor.
2 Now tip back on your bottom and lift your feet off the floor.
3 Aim to reach your hands out in front of you and maintain your balance by strongly contracting your abdominals. If you can't straighten your legs, then just keep them bent but lifted off the floor.
4 Touch your feet back to the floor in between each repetition to regain the start position.

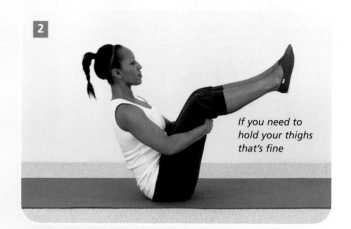

If you need to hold your thighs that's fine

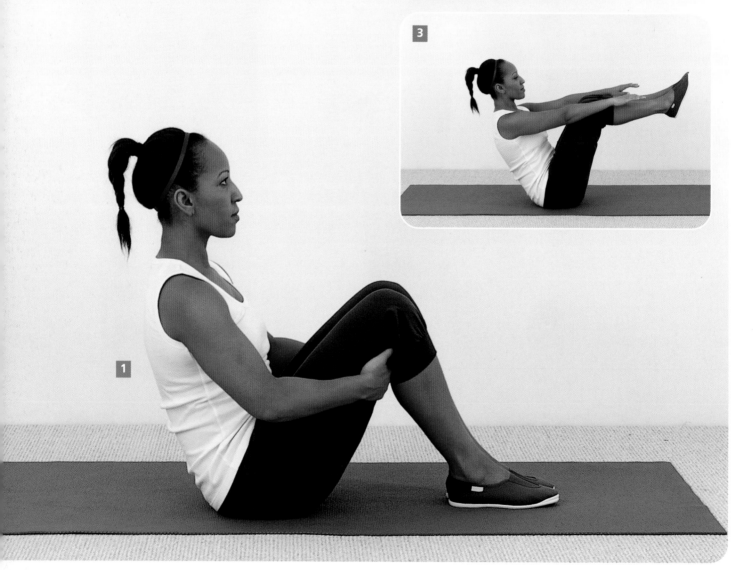

HYPEREXTENSION

As well as working on strengthening and pulling in to flatten your abdominal muscles, you also need to think about another key part of your "core"—and that is your back muscles. During pregnancy, your back muscles were under pressure carrying extra weight that pulled your center of gravity forward, and your spinal joints were affected by the hormone, relaxin, which softens the supporting ligaments. In addition to this, the sacro-iliac joints (where the back of the pelvis joins the spine) are often vulnerable to injury after pregnancy so strengthening the muscles that support the spine is very important.

This exercise and its variations will help strengthen the erector spinae muscles that run either side of the vertebrae and help with movement of the spine. Learning to use these muscles in conjunction with your abdominals will mean your whole core area is better supported and less prone to strains and pains.

BEGINNER'S POSE

1 Lie prone (on your front) with your hands clasped behind your back and your forehead on the floor.
2 Gently lift up your head and chest as you leave your legs, relaxed, on the floor. You will feel the back muscle working as you lift.

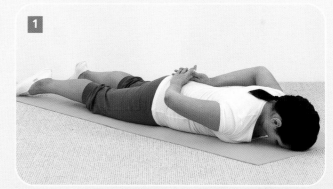

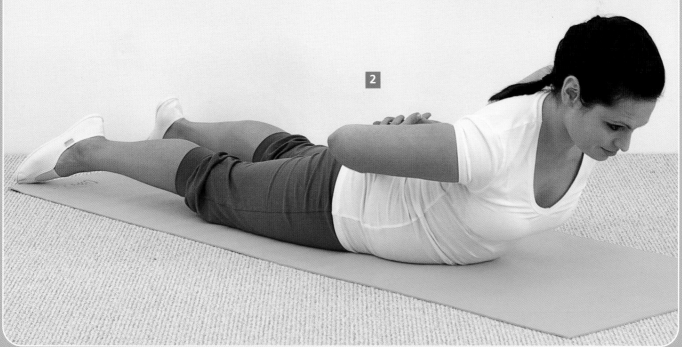

VARIATIONS

SHOULDER HYPE

REPS **8** INTENSITY **moderate**

This can be done from week 3

1 Lie prone with your hands touching your shoulders.

2 Now lift your upper body off the floor, contracting your back muscles to rise as high as you can.

3 With control, lower your upper body to the floor and repeat.

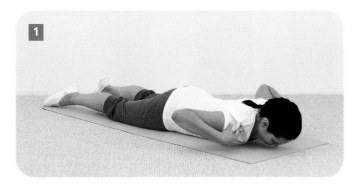

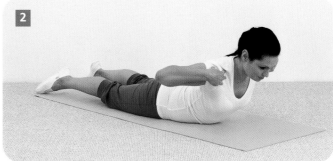

BALL ARCH

REPS **10** INTENSITY **moderate**

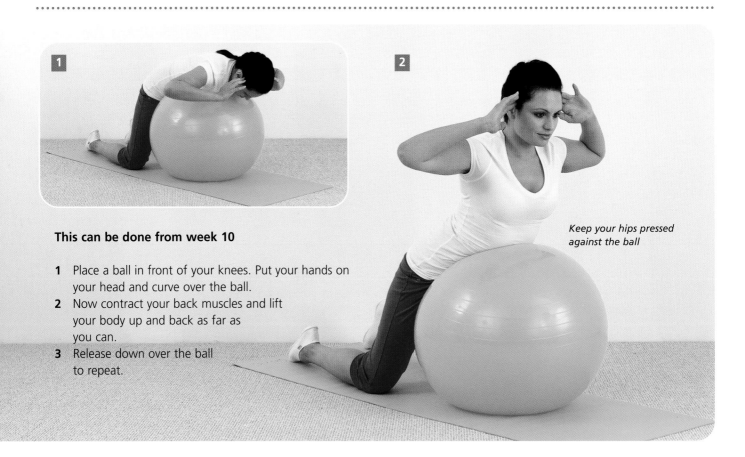

This can be done from week 10

1 Place a ball in front of your knees. Put your hands on your head and curve over the ball.

2 Now contract your back muscles and lift your body up and back as far as you can.

3 Release down over the ball to repeat.

Keep your hips pressed against the ball

STRAIGHT ARM BALL ARCH

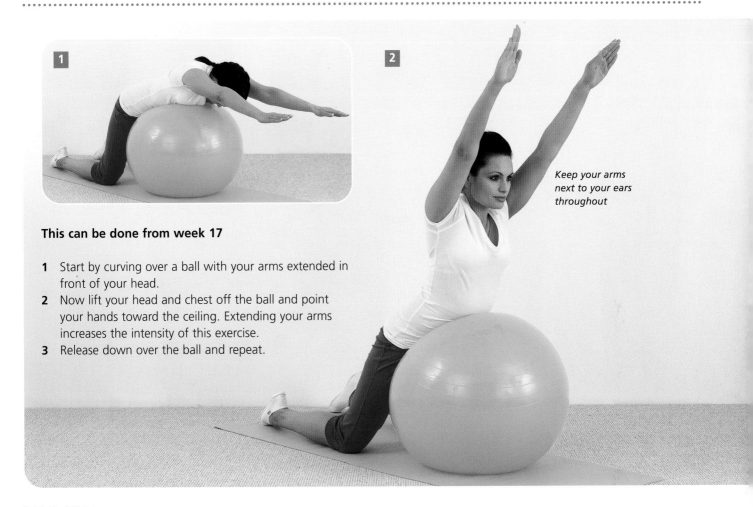

Keep your arms next to your ears throughout

This can be done from week 17

1 Start by curving over a ball with your arms extended in front of your head.
2 Now lift your head and chest off the ball and point your hands toward the ceiling. Extending your arms increases the intensity of this exercise.
3 Release down over the ball and repeat.

LEG FLY

This can be done from week 24

1 Lie on the floor with your forehead resting on your hands.

2 Now extend through your toes to straighten your legs and then use this energy to lift them off the floor as high as you can.
3 Lower down to repeat.

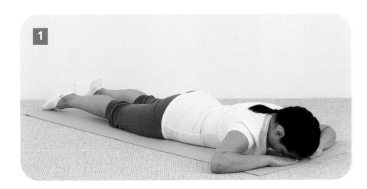

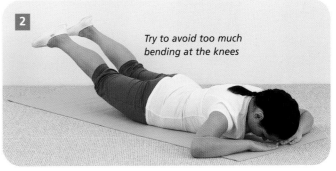

Try to avoid too much bending at the knees

DOLPHIN LIFT

This can be done from week 31

1. Lie face down on the floor with your arms and legs extended.
2. Now raise your right arm and left leg off the floor simultaneously and then lower.
3. Repeat with your left arm and right leg.

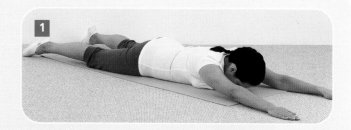

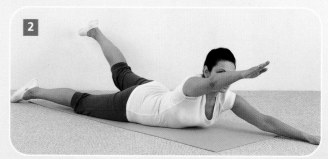

You are working the erector spinae muscles that run alongside the spine

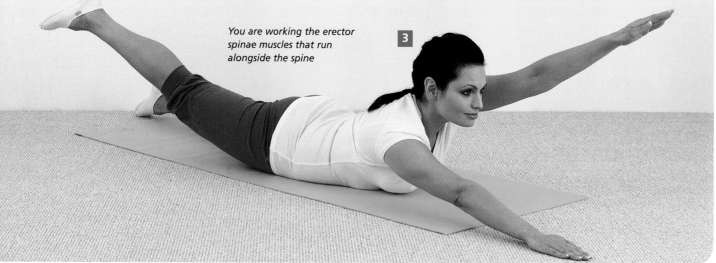

QUAD HYPE   REPS **4 on each side** INTENSITY **moderate**

This can be done from week 35

- Lie on your front and come up on one elbow. Now reach behind with your other hand to take hold of the foot on that side. Work your back muscles more by holding onto the foot and trying to lift your chest even higher off the floor. Repeat on other side.

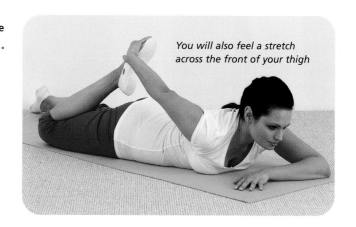

You will also feel a stretch across the front of your thigh

ROLL DOWN

This set of exercises is all about using your spine as a "flexible whole." Flexing and extending areas of the spine is good for back health as movement in this area produces warmth and has an "oiling" effect on the joints of the vertebral column. Think of the pelvis as connected to the spine so that it becomes part of the movement and, as you move, curving your spine and pelvis will also work other areas of the abdomen. The exercise will be more fun with your baby at your feet.

REPS **4–5 times until smooth**
INTENSITY **moderate**

BASIC ROLL DOWN

1 Start by standing upright with your knees slightly bent.
2 Now slowly start to curl your body over, starting by dropping your head.
3 Let your head pull your spine into a forward curl.
4 Try to let your arms just hang and feel your spine curving over, almost vertebra by vertebra.
5 Eventually, with more bending of the knees, you will have curled over far enough for your hands to be near the floor (or to touch your baby).
6 When you are down far enough, lift your head and slowly uncurl from your lower spine through your middle back, pulling in your abdominals and keeping your head hanging until you have uncurled at the neck. Finish by standing as tall as you can.

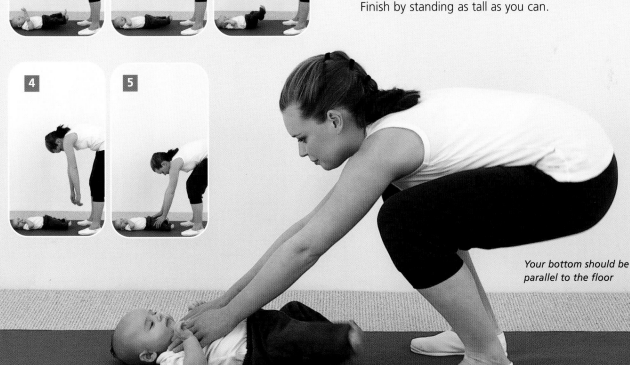

Your bottom should be parallel to the floor

VARIATIONS

OBLIQUE SHRUG

REPS **5 on each side** INTENSITY **light**

This can be done from week 2

1 Lie on your back with your arms out to the side.

2 Now contract your side abdominal muscles (the obliques) and try to bring your right shoulder closer to your right hip, shortening the distance between these two joints.

3 Release and contract on the other side.

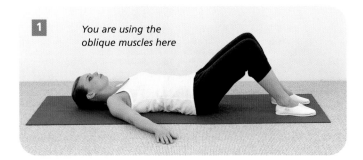

You are using the oblique muscles here

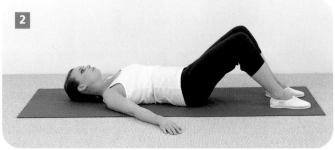

HIP HITCH

REPS **8 on each side** INTENSITY **light**

This can be done from week 4

1 Sit on a ball and place your weight equally on both buttocks and both feet.

2 Now contract your abdominal muscles (the obliques) on one side and bring this hip nearer your shoulder.

3 Repeat this move on the other side.

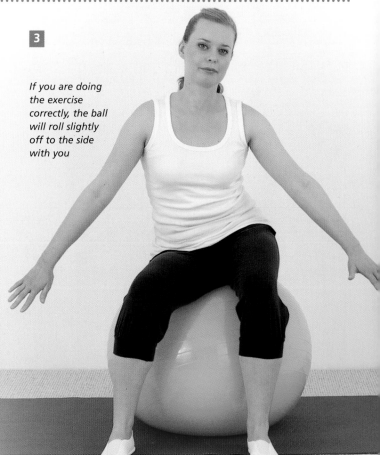

If you are doing the exercise correctly, the ball will roll slightly off to the side with you

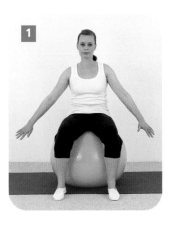

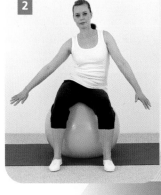

STRAIGHT ARM ROLL DOWN

This can be done from week 8

1 Start sitting on the floor with your knees bent and arms out in front of you.
2 Slowly roll your back down toward the floor.
3 Aim to curve your spine slowly and gradually (this is where the abdominal work comes in).
4 Really try to feel as though you are lowering your spine onto the floor link by link, vertebra by vertebra.
5 Finish supine on the floor. Roll over on to your side and push yourself back up to sitting to begin the roll down again.

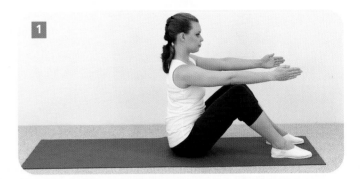

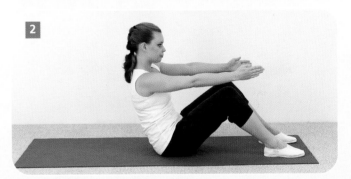

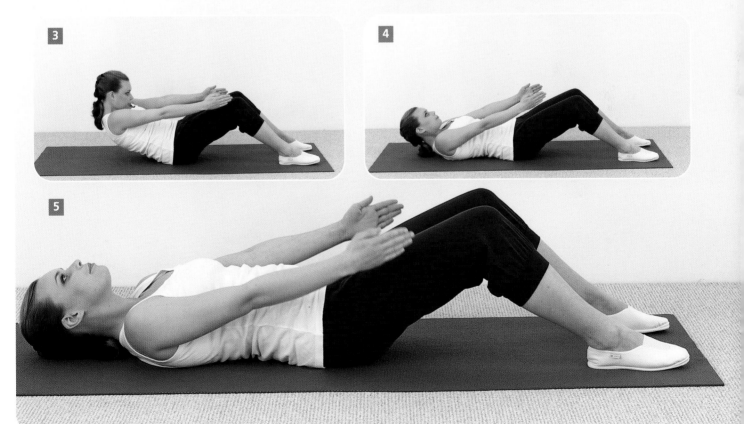

CROSS YOUR HEART

REPS **3–4** INTENSITY **moderate**

This can be done from week 13

1. Sit up straight with your arms crossed on your chest, knees bent, and your feet flat on the floor.
2. Slowly roll down, vertebra by vertebra.
3. Finish supine on the floor then roll over onto your side and push yourself back up to sitting to begin the roll down again.

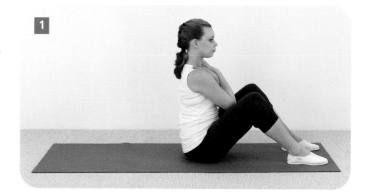

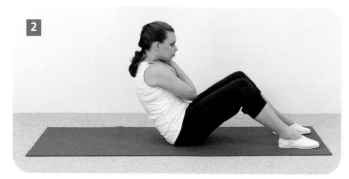

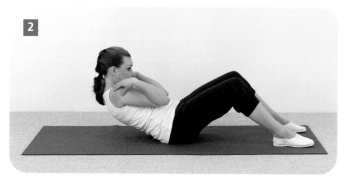

SHOULDER SHRUG ROLL

REPS **3–4** INTENSITY **moderate**

This can be done from week 16

1. Start by sitting with knees bent and hands touching your shoulders.
2. Roll down, curving your upper back, and slowly lowering each part of your spine onto the floor.
3. Keep curving your spine until you are flat on the floor, then roll over onto your side and push yourself back up to sitting to begin the roll down again.

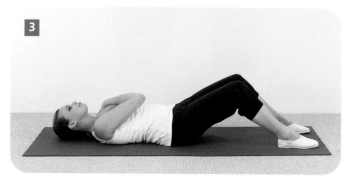

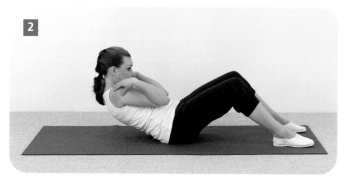

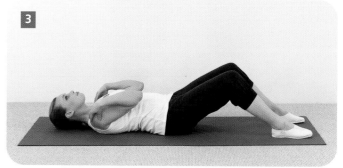

NECKLACE ROLL DOWN

REPS 3–4 INTENSITY moderate

This can be done from week 21

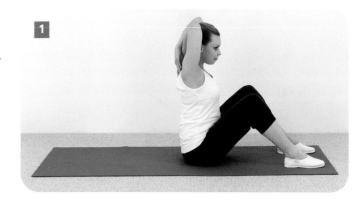

1 Start in a sitting position with both arms behind your head, each hand touching the opposite shoulder blade.
2 Slowly roll down, curving your spine.
3 Finish by lying flat on the floor; resist the urge to just flop straight down!
4 When you're ready to come up, take a deep breath, roll over onto your side, and push yourself back up to sitting.

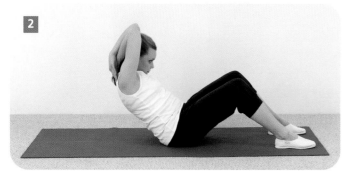

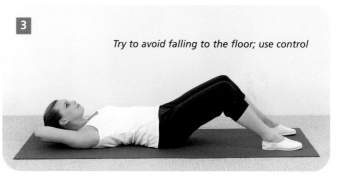

Try to avoid falling to the floor; use control

HIP ARCH

REPS/TIME 6–8 slow roll ups INTENSITY moderate

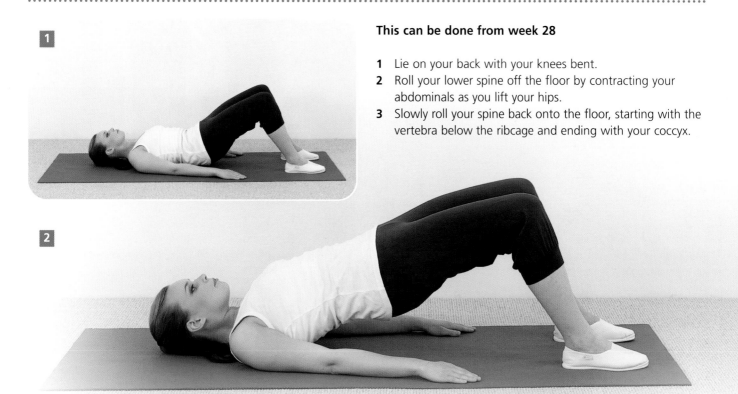

This can be done from week 28

1 Lie on your back with your knees bent.
2 Roll your lower spine off the floor by contracting your abdominals as you lift your hips.
3 Slowly roll your spine back onto the floor, starting with the vertebra below the ribcage and ending with your coccyx.

HIP ARCH & PULSE

This can be done from week 34

1 Lie flat on your back with your knees bent.
2 Curve your lower spine off the floor to lift your hips high up in the air (you'll feel your buttock muscles working too!).
3 Now pulse your hips up and down at least 20 times then slowly lower your spine back onto the floor. Repeat from step 2.

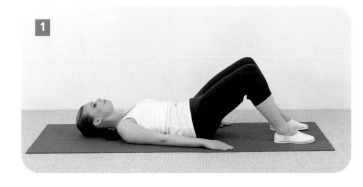

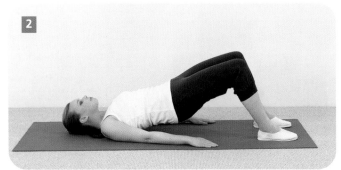

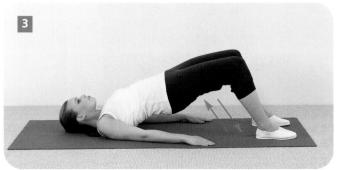

BABY HILLTOP

REPS **10–12** INTENSITY **moderate**

This can be done from week 38

1 Lie on your back with your knees bent and place your baby comfortably across your hips. Hold him/her in place with your hands.
2 Now curve your lower spine off the floor and lift, taking your baby's weight with you. From this position, you can even do a few pulses to keep him/her entertained!
3 Slowly lower your hips (holding onto your baby) to the floor. Repeat from step 2.

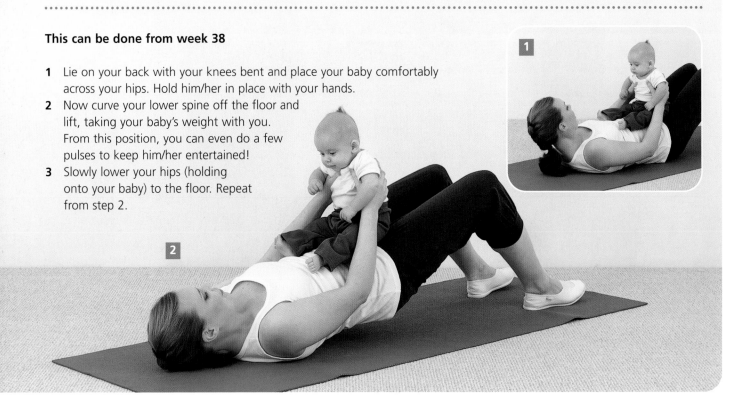

PRESS UPS

Press ups are a perfect full-body exercise. They work the chest and arm muscles as well as the abdominals and, in the full version, they work the buttocks, too.

There are different stages of press up that can be done until you build enough strength to do a full position press up. Each time you change your arms or body position, you will be working different muscles. For example, the tri press (from week 14) focuses tension on the triceps muscle at the back of the arms.

Always aim to keep your mid back straight so there is no dipping of the hips toward the floor. This will encourage a flat stomach as you engage your transverse muscles.

ALL FOURS POSITION

REPS **10**
INTENSITY **moderate**

1 Start on all fours keeping more of your weight on your hands than on your knees.
2 Bend your arms to the side and lower your nose until it almost touches the floor.
3 Straighten your arms to come up. Repeat from step 2.

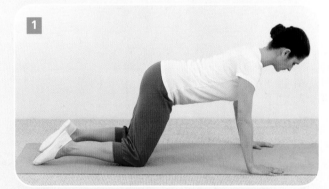

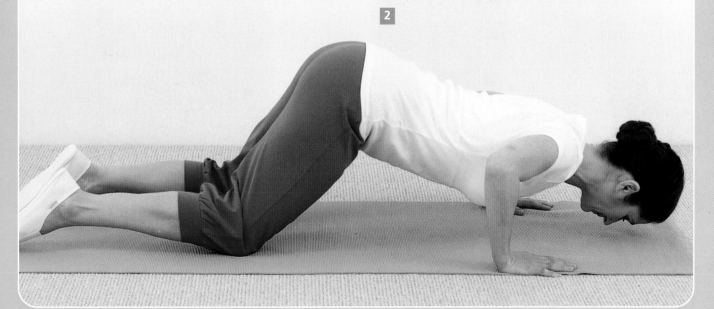

VARIATIONS

3/4 PRESS UP

This can be done from week 2

1 Start on all fours, then lean forward until your weight is mainly on your arms and bend and cross your legs. Make sure there is a straight line from your hips to your shoulders and your bottom is not sticking up.

2 Slowly bend your arms, lowering your entire body until your nose and hips are just off the floor.

3 Straighten your arms to lift up and repeat.

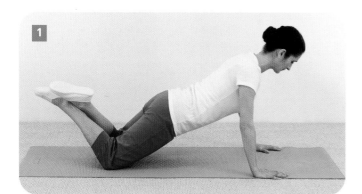

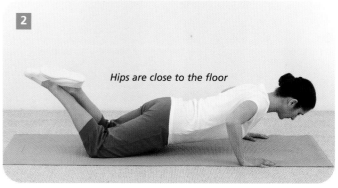

Hips are close to the floor

WIDE ARM PRESS UP

This can be done from week 7

1 Start on all fours, extending your arms out to the sides in a "wide" stance and lean forward until your weight is mainly on your arms. Bend and cross your legs.

2 Slowly lower your whole body down until it is just off the floor and then straighten your arms to lift again.

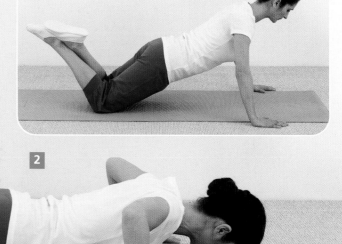

This variation focuses the intensity on your chest muscles

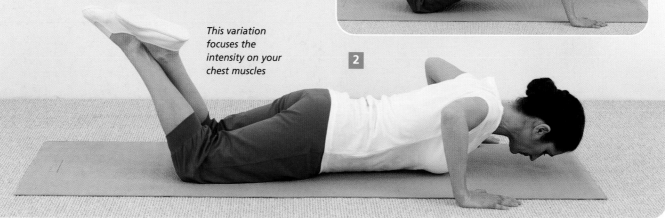

UNEVEN ARM PRESS

This can be done from week 12

1   Start in the ¾ position (see opposite page).

2   Place one hand in front of the other, then lower your whole body until it is just off the floor.

3   Extend your arms to come back up. Repeat with the other hand in front.

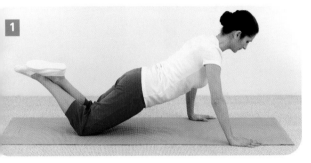

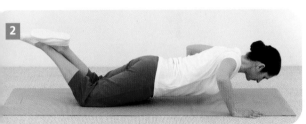

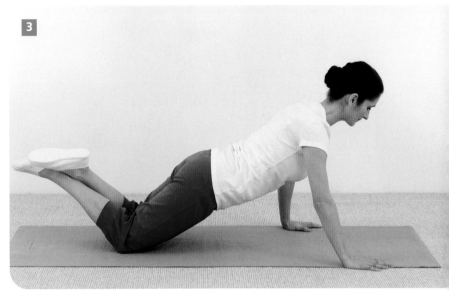

TRI PRESS

This can be done from week 14

1   Start in the ¾ position (see opposite page) but tuck your arms tight into the sides of your ribcage as you lower your body. Keep your arms next to your body (not out to the side) with your elbows in line with your shoulders.

2   When you reach the lowest point, check again that your arms are pressed close to your ribcage with your elbows behind you.

3   Extend your arms to start over again.

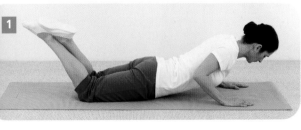

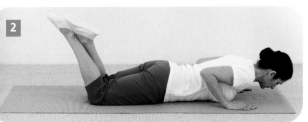

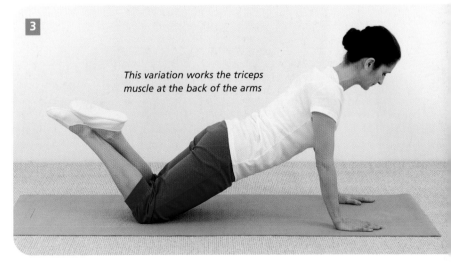

This variation works the triceps muscle at the back of the arms

BALL PRESS

This can be done from week 30

1 Start by leaning forward over a ball and walking your hands out in front of you until your hips are balanced on the ball. Contract your abdominals firmly to keep your position stable.

2 Bend your arms until your nose is just off the floor. To make this exercise more challenging, roll the ball further backward with your feet so that your hips are not resting on it.

3 Once you have completed your reps, walk your hands backward, carefully rolling the ball underneath your hips. Lower your legs to the floor to stand up off the ball.

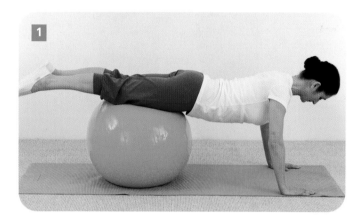

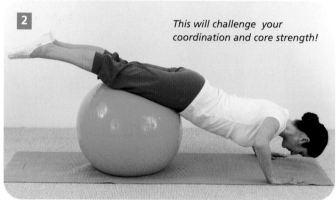

This will challenge your coordination and core strength!

FULL PRESS UP

This can be done from week 34

1 Start with your toes and hands on the floor, and your abdominal muscles tensed to support your straight spine.

2 Maintaining a straight back, lower your body, arms bent at the elbows, until you are almost touching the floor.

3 To press back up, straighten your arms.

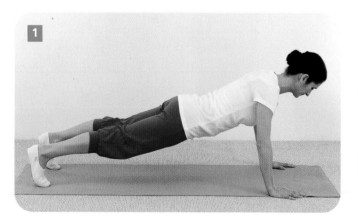

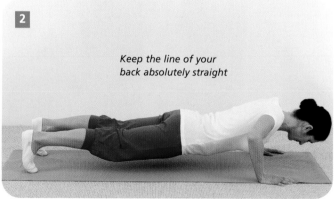

Keep the line of your back absolutely straight

THIGH TONERS

Arm and leg strength play a key part in keeping your body moving easily and you'll need strong arms and legs because you have an increasingly heavy baby to lift! Some women store fat around their thigh area during pregnancy and while exercises can't reduce fat in specific areas, toning the thigh and buttock muscles will make this area look and feel much better.

The outer and inner thigh muscles (the abductors and adductors) often get less toning than the quadriceps and hamstrings (on the front and back of thigh) so this series of exercises will target and shape your outer and inner thighs and your buttock muscles.

BASIC ALL FOURS

• Get down on your hands and knees making sure you support your weight equally on them. Draw your belly up toward your spine but don't suck it up completely—feel some tension in the abdominal area so that you know those muscles are working.

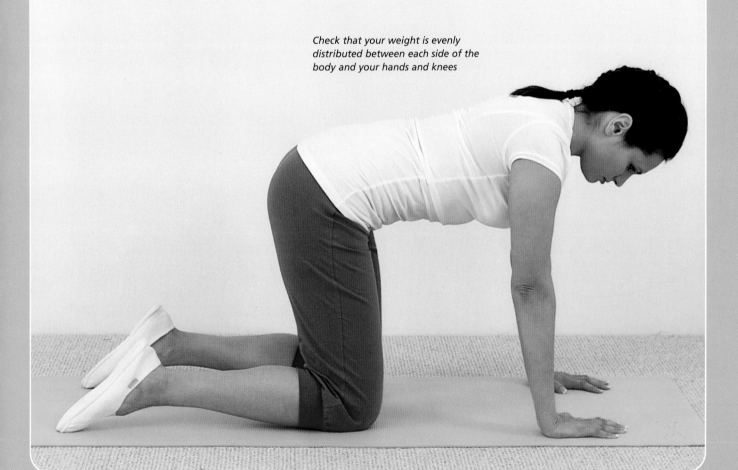

Check that your weight is evenly distributed between each side of the body and your hands and knees

VARIATIONS

BACK KICK

This can be done from week 7

1 Start on all fours then extend your right leg out behind you.
2 Lift this leg off the floor as high as you can.

3 Touch the foot back down to the floor and then lift to repeat.
4 After 10 reps, bend your right leg in and extend your left leg. Repeat from step 2.

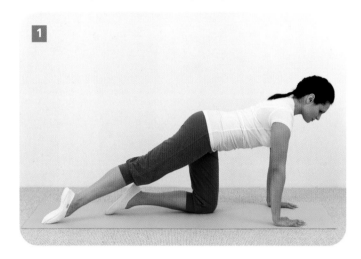

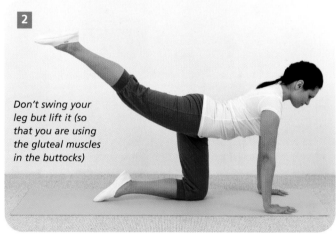

Don't swing your leg but lift it (so that you are using the gluteal muscles in the buttocks)

DONKEY LIFT

REPS **10 on each leg** INTENSITY **moderate**

This can be done from week 13

1 Start on all fours, pulling up your abdominal area.

2 Lift one leg (keeping the knee bent) directly out to the side and hold briefly.
3 Lower your leg and repeat for 10 reps. Then lift your other leg and repeat from step 2.

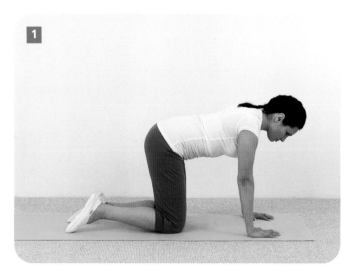

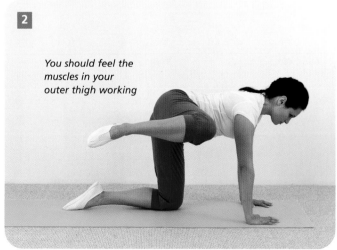

You should feel the muscles in your outer thigh working

DONKEY KICK

This can be done from week 24

1 Start on all fours with your weight spread equally on your hands and knees and your abdominals tightened.
2 Now lift one bent leg out to the side at approximately hip height.
3 Extend the leg, keeping it at the same height off the floor.
4 Bend the leg back in again (as photo 2) and lower it down to the floor to reach the start position. When you've done your 10 reps, repeat from step 2 with your other leg.

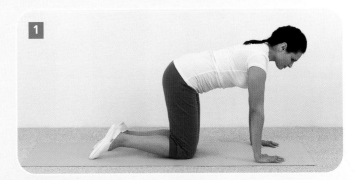

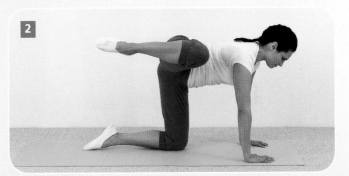

Be sure to keep your leg at hip height from the floor as you extend out to the side

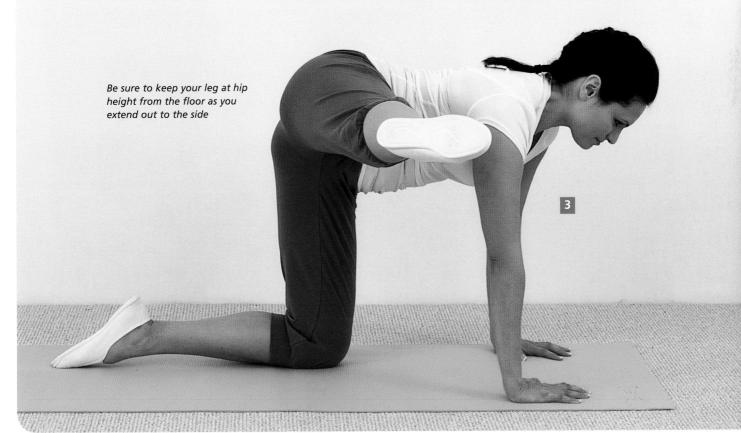

CIRCLES

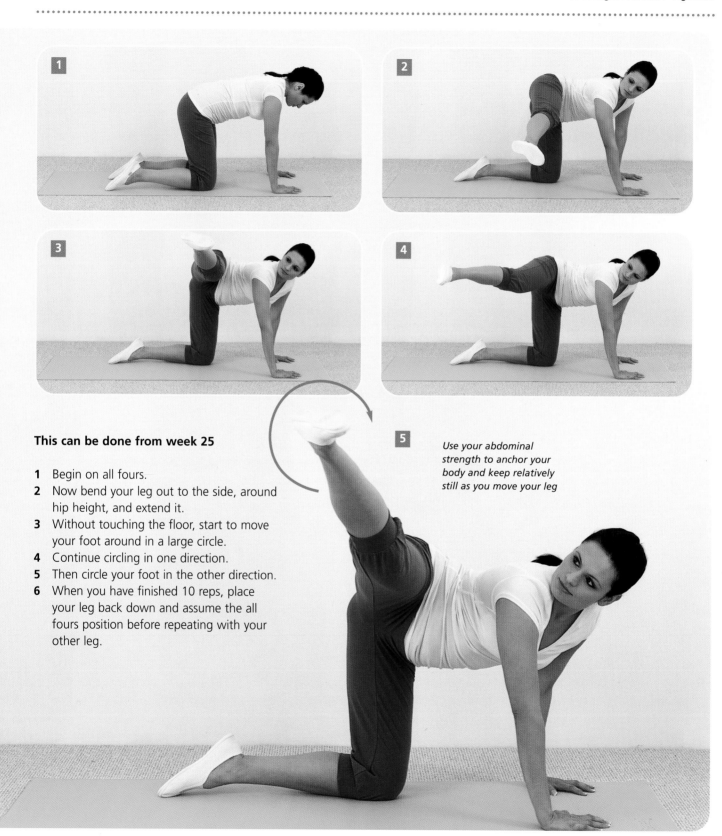

This can be done from week 25

1 Begin on all fours.
2 Now bend your leg out to the side, around hip height, and extend it.
3 Without touching the floor, start to move your foot around in a large circle.
4 Continue circling in one direction.
5 Then circle your foot in the other direction.
6 When you have finished 10 reps, place your leg back down and assume the all fours position before repeating with your other leg.

Use your abdominal strength to anchor your body and keep relatively still as you move your leg

LEG SWING

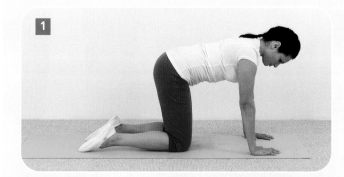

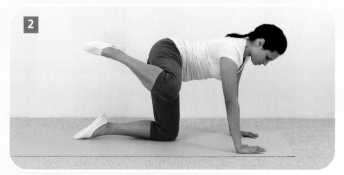

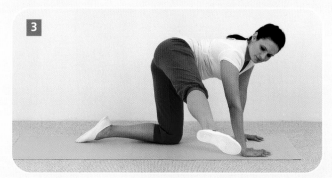

This can be done from week 32

1 Start on all fours.
2 Now lift one leg and bend it so it is at hip height.
3 Extend the leg to the side.
4 Then, keeping your leg raised, swing it to the back and lift it up behind you as far as you can.
5 Lower the leg back down to hip height as in step 2 then extend it out and back to the side; repeat until you've finished all the reps on one leg. .
6 Replace the leg on the floor and repeat with the other leg.

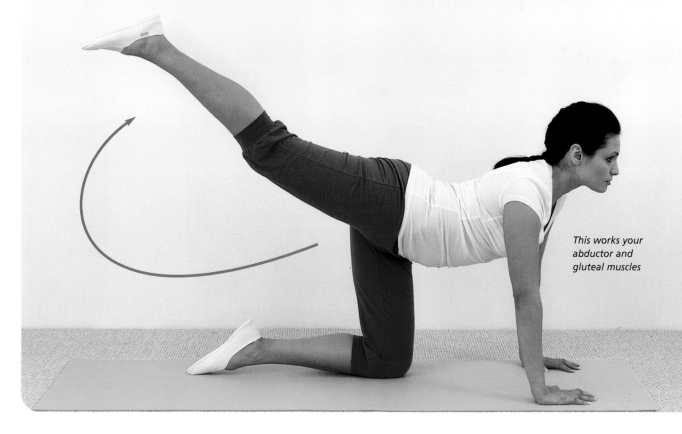

This works your abductor and gluteal muscles

SQUAT

The squat is a great exercise for strengthening and toning the muscles of the lower body. As you bend and straighten in this exercise, you are using the major muscles of the thighs including the quadriceps (front of thigh) the hamstrings (back of thigh), and bottom (gluteus maximus).

The key with this exercise (and all its variations) is to keep your body, from your hips to your shoulders, in a straight line and to keep your weight over your heels as you lower.

REPS **10**
INTENSITY **light**

BASIC SQUAT

1   Start by standing tall; your shoulders should be pulled back and down, your ribcage lifted off your waist, and your coccyx (tail bone) should pull toward the floor.
2   Now press your bottom out behind you as you lower downward, bending your knees. Reach your arms out in front to balance yourself.
3   To come up, straighten your knees, keeping your back straight and pressing your hips forward.

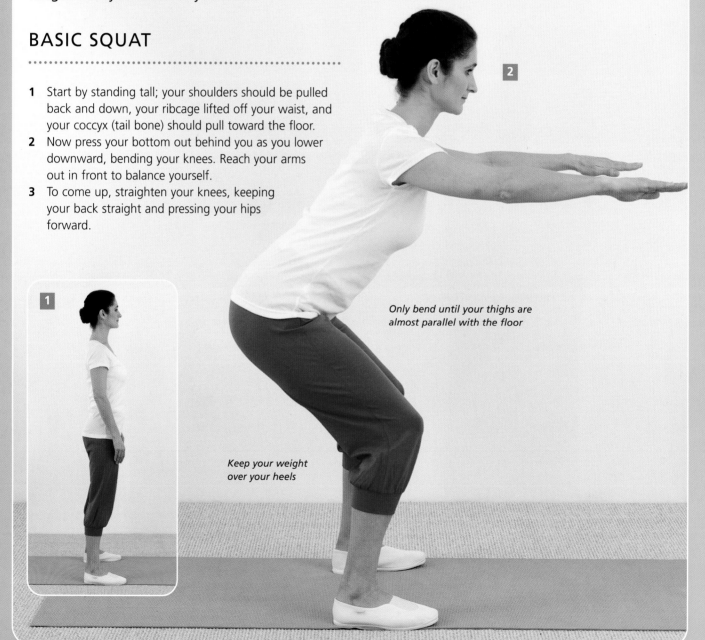

Only bend until your thighs are almost parallel with the floor

Keep your weight over your heels

VARIATIONS

SQUAT WITH BICEP CURL

REPS **10** INTENSITY **light**

This can be done from week 4

1 Begin in the start position: shoulders pulled back and down, ribcage lifted off your waist, and your coccyx pulling toward the floor.
2 Bend your knees and lower into the squat position. As you do this, contract your biceps, bending your arms, and bring your fists toward you.
3 Lower your arms, stand tall, and repeat from step 2.

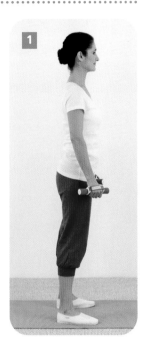

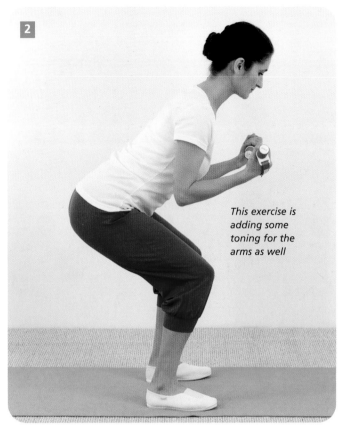

This exercise is adding some toning for the arms as well

PRISONER SQUAT

REPS **10** INTENSITY **moderate**

This can be done from week 19

1 Stand tall and place your hands behind your head.
2 Lower your bottom behind you and toward the floor and bend your knees, but keep your upper body lifted. Try and go slightly lower than you have done on previous weeks.
3 When you have bent your legs as far as is manageable, straighten your knees and press your hips forward to come up.

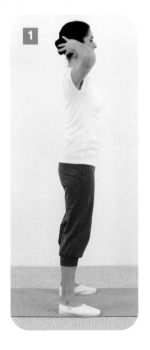

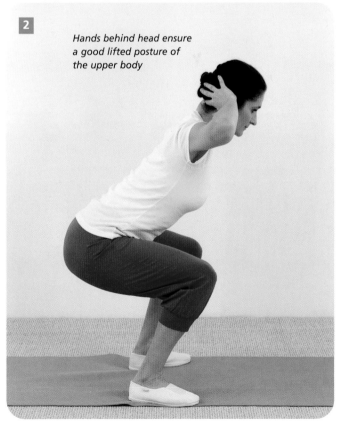

Hands behind head ensure a good lifted posture of the upper body

BARBELL SQUAT

REPS **12 (hold for 1–2 seconds)** INTENSITY **moderate**

This can be done from week 29

1 Begin by lifting up the barbell under your chin.
2 From here, lift the bar up and over your head and place it on the muscular part of your upper back.
3 Bend your knees and lower your bottom back and down but keep your upper body lifted and supporting the bar. Hold for 1–2 seconds.
4 To come up, press your hips forward and straighten your legs.

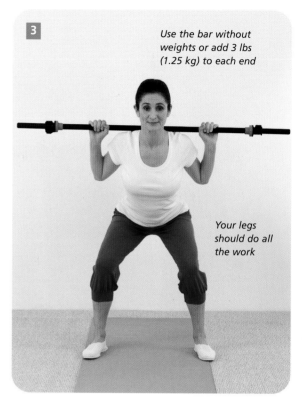

Use the bar without weights or add 3 lbs (1.25 kg) to each end

Your legs should do all the work

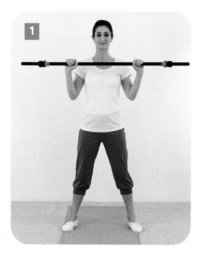

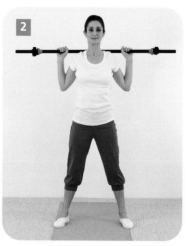

ONE LEG SQUAT

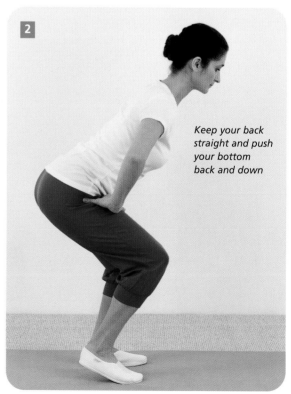

REPS **8 on each leg** INTENSITY **vigorous**

This can be done from week 38

1 Stand on your left foot with the toe of your right foot just touching the floor to balance you.
2 Now squat down, with all your weight on your left leg; your right foot should just touch the floor for balance.
3 Straighten your left leg to come back to the starting position and then repeat with your right leg.

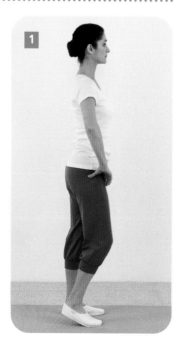

Keep your back straight and push your bottom back and down

LUNGE

REPS **8 on each leg**
INTENSITY **moderate**

Even though you will often see it performed in the gym and on DVDs, the lunge is quite an advanced move and you need to get it right. As you lower and rise, it is important to keep your body going up and down on a purely vertical axis; do not lurch forward and backward as this will put pressure on your knee (don't forget your ligaments are still soft from the action of pregnancy hormones).

When you have mastered this move, you will feel it really working your leg muscles, particularly your front thigh muscles (quadriceps), and those in the back of your legs and calves (hamstrings and gastrocnemius).

BASIC LUNGE

- Step forward into a wide split step so that your back heel is lifted. Place your hands on your hips, pull your abdominals in toward your spine, and lift your ribcage up off your waist. Lower yourself down until your back and front legs are bent at right angles. Contract your abdominals to help you balance. Slowly straighten both legs to come up with control. Repeat the sequence with your other leg.

Keep your shoulders pulled back and down

Your front knee should not go beyond your foot

Bend your legs so that your back knee goes directly toward the floor

Your weight should be between your two feet so that as you bend, you feel both your back leg and front leg working

VARIATIONS

BACK STEP LUNGE

REPS **8 on each leg** INTENSITY **moderate**

This can be done from week 3

1 Start in a straight, lifted position with your hands on your hips. Your abdominals should be pulled in toward your spine and your ribcage lifted up off your waist.

2 Step forward on your left leg into a wide split step so that your back heel is lifted.

3 Reach your right leg behind you and lower into the lunge. Stay for 2 seconds then bring your right leg back in as you rise up to a straight lifted position.

4 Repeat, stepping forward on your right leg.

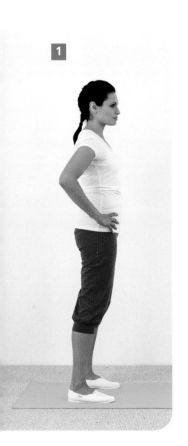

1

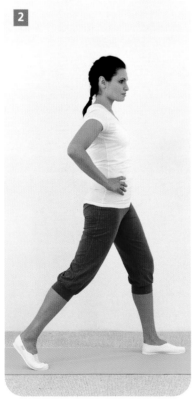

2

3

Aim to keep your body as stable as possible by contracting your abdominals

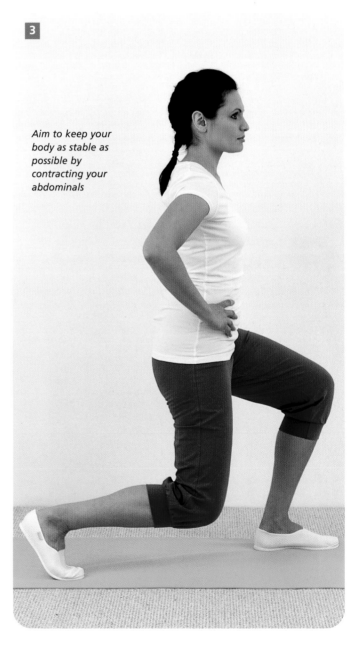

FORWARD STEP LUNGE

REPS **10 on each leg** INTENSITY **moderate**

This can be done from week 22

1 From a lifted, standing position, with your weights at hip height, take a wide step forward.
2 Lower yourself into the lunge position (front leg at 90 degrees) while at the same time bringing the weights up to your chest.
3 Straighten your arms and push back off your front foot to come back to two feet and then repeat on the other leg.

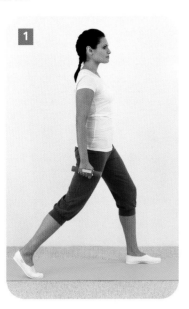

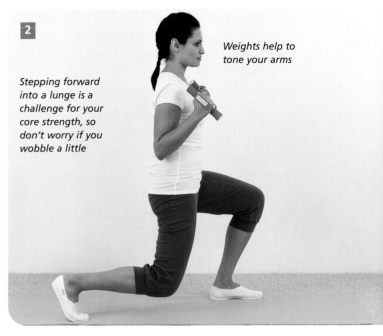

Weights help to tone your arms

Stepping forward into a lunge is a challenge for your core strength, so don't worry if you wobble a little

LEAP LUNGE

REPS **8 on each leg** INTENSITY **vigorous**

This can be done from week 36

1 Step forward (or back) into the lunge position and bend low preparing to spring into the air. Take your arms back.
2 Leap up, swing your arms forward, and while you are airborne, swap your legs so that you land with the opposite leg in front.
3 On landing, really bend your legs to absorb the impact of your jump.
4 Repeat steps 1 to 3 starting off with the other leg in front.

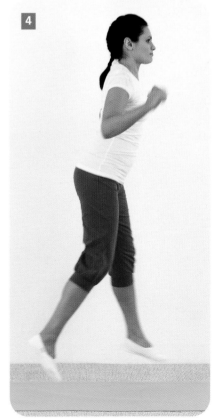

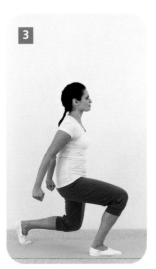

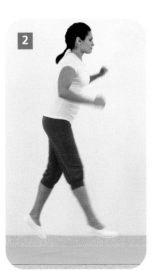

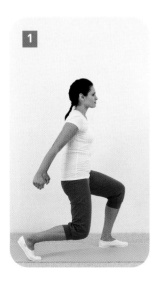

BODY STRETCH

REPS/TIME 1–2
(hold for 5 seconds)
INTENSITY light

Stretching at the end of a muscle toning session is necessary for several reasons. Stretching and moving more gently help slow the blood flow down gradually and lengthen the muscles back to their original pre-exercise length. Time spent stationary at the end of a workout may help the body adjust and assimilate the changes that have occurred due to the demands of the workout.

This stretch and its variations will loosen and stretch out the areas of your body so that your muscles don't remain contracted but are lengthened and given time to recover. This will hopefully leave you feeling refreshed and revitalized.

FULL BODY STRETCH

- Lie supine with your hands above your head and legs stretched out straight. Breathe in, and as you exhale, stretch your hands away from your feet as much as you can. Your whole body will be in tension as you st-r-e-t-ch. Then release and fully relax.

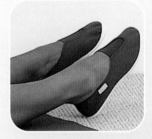

On the stretch, both your hands and feet should reach out from your body

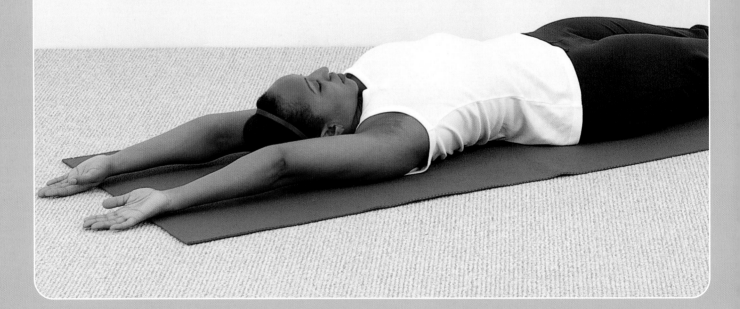

SIDE STRETCH

This can be done from week 3

1 Lie on your back and spread your arms out to the side.
2 Now lift both knees up to your chest, keeping your feet together.
3 Using your abdominals to control the movement, slowly swing your knees over to one side and let them rest on the floor.
4 Lift your knees and slowly swing them to the other side, letting them rest on the floor before raising them to chest height and then placing them flat on the floor.

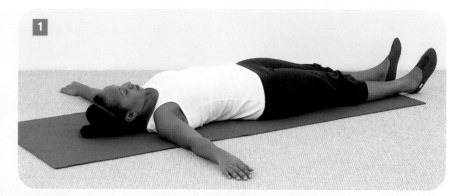

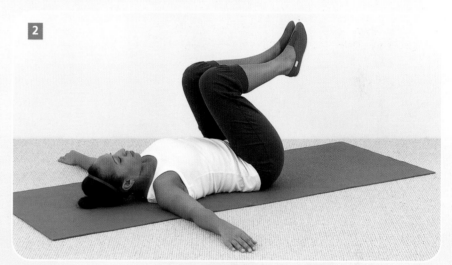

You should feel a pleasant stretch across your lower back

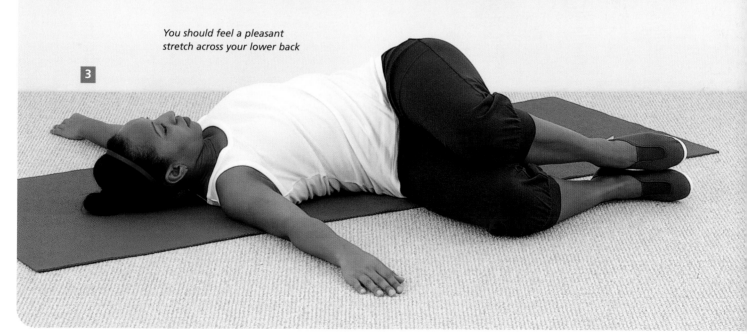

RAISED LEG STRETCH

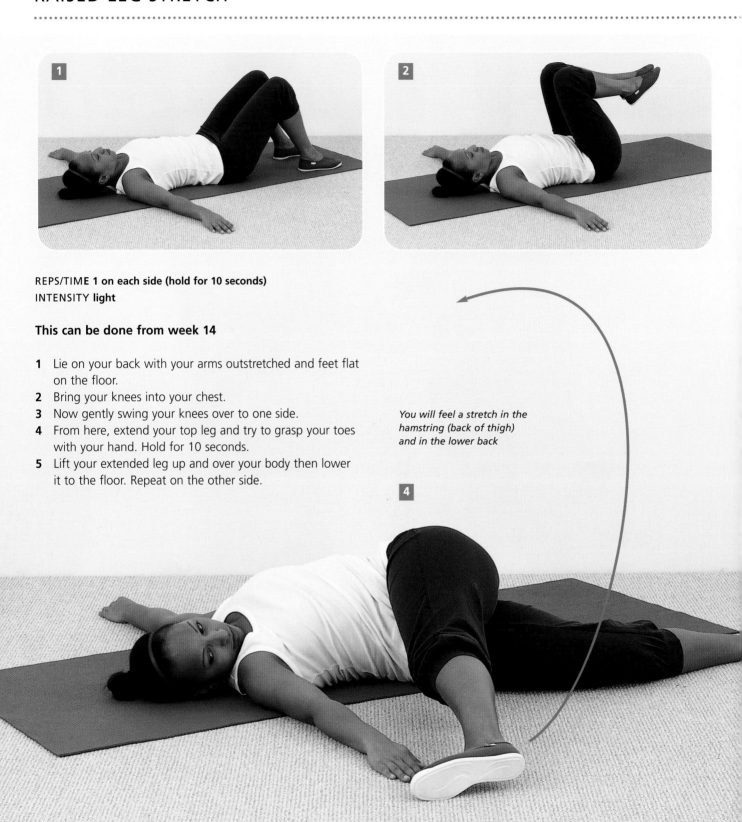

REPS/TIME **1 on each side (hold for 10 seconds)**
INTENSITY **light**

This can be done from week 14

1 Lie on your back with your arms outstretched and feet flat
   on the floor.
2 Bring your knees into your chest.
3 Now gently swing your knees over to one side.
4 From here, extend your top leg and try to grasp your toes
   with your hand. Hold for 10 seconds.
5 Lift your extended leg up and over your body then lower
   it to the floor. Repeat on the other side.

*You will feel a stretch in the
hamstring (back of thigh)
and in the lower back*

SITTING TWIST

REPS/TIME 1 on each side (hold for 10 seconds)
INTENSITY light

This can be done from week 29

1 Sit upright, with your back straight and your legs flat out in front of you.
2 Now bend your right knee, bringing your right foot close to your body. Twist your torso toward your right knee, wrapping your left hand around it. Turn your head and upper body to complete the stretch, twisting as far around as you can.
3 Release and repeat the stretch on the other side.

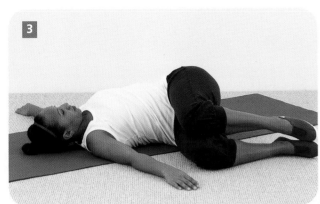

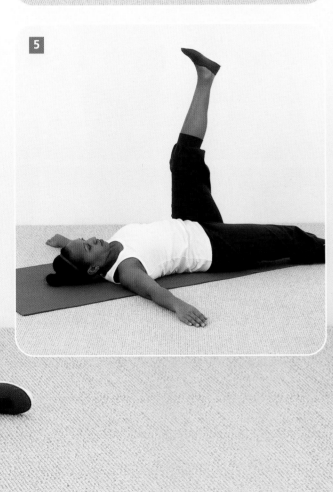

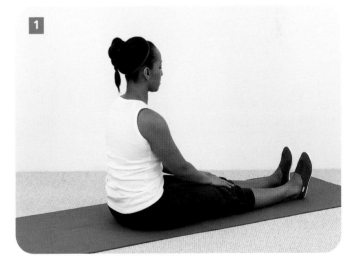

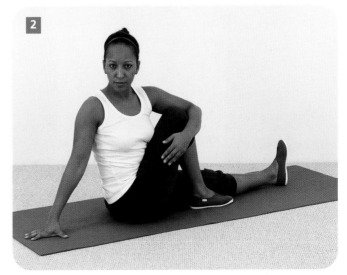

COOL DOWN

For each exercise
REPS/TIME 1–2 (hold for 10–15 seconds with a feeling of mild tension)

TRI & LUNGE

Step your left leg in front of you and bend both knees. Now transfer your weight slightly onto your back foot and tilt your back hip up slightly (by contracting your lower abdominals) so that you feel a stretch on the front of that hip. At the same time, reach your right arm up and behind you; use your other hand to press the arm back so that you feel a stretch (of the triceps muscle) at the back of your right arm. Hold, then repeat on the other side.

You will feel a stretch across the front of your hips

LINK & REACH

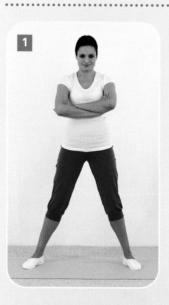 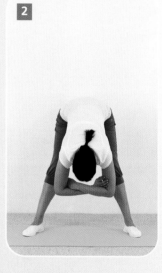

1 Stand tall and cross your arms. Engage your abdominals so that your core is supported.
  2 Very gently, start to lean forward and drop your folded arms toward the floor. You should feel a stretch on the back of your thigns (hamstrings). If there is any discomfort in your lower back, unfold your arms and place your hands on your thighs or shins for support. Hold then release your arms to curl slowly back up.

SIDE REACH

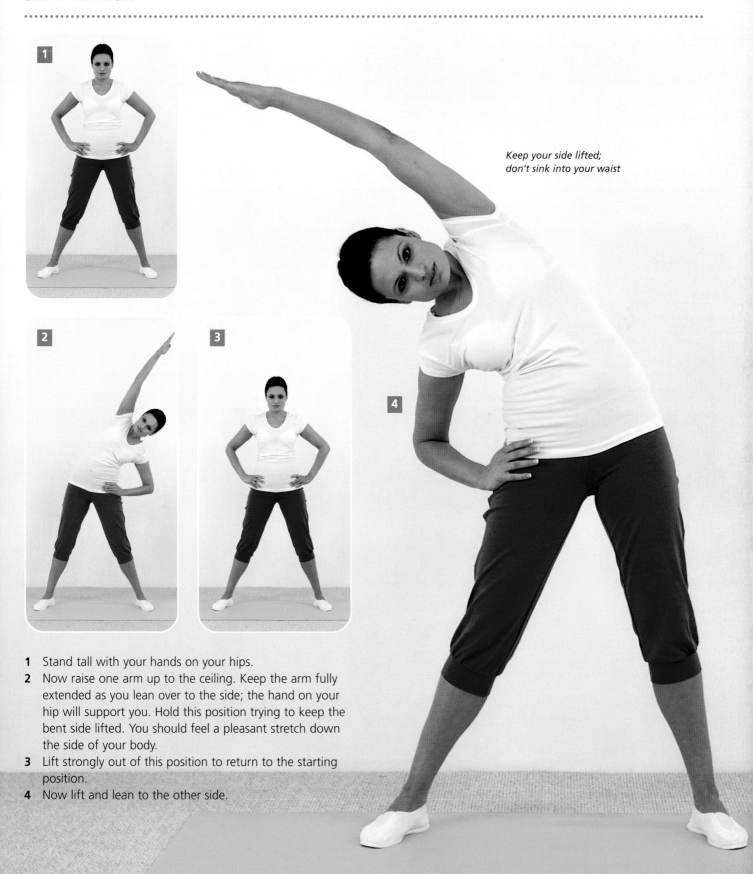

Keep your side lifted; don't sink into your waist

1 Stand tall with your hands on your hips.
2 Now raise one arm up to the ceiling. Keep the arm fully extended as you lean over to the side; the hand on your hip will support you. Hold this position trying to keep the bent side lifted. You should feel a pleasant stretch down the side of your body.
3 Lift strongly out of this position to return to the starting position.
4 Now lift and lean to the other side.

YOUR EXERCISE DIARY

1   2   3   4

WEEKS 1–4 The pages that follow allow you to keep track of your progress from the first week you exercise until you have shifted all your pregnancy weight gain and toned and shaped your body. Use this space to record your own goals (which may differ from those of the program), whether you've completed some or all of that week's program, and what you do on the days when you don't "work out."

MY GOALS				
MONDAY				
TUESDAY				
WEDNESDAY				
THURSDAY				
FRIDAY				
SATURDAY				
SUNDAY				

WEEKS 5–8 You're well into the program and, although there may be very little so far to show for all your work, rest assured that it is paying off. Your cardiovascular fitness is undoubtedly improving and as time goes by you'll find—even if your nights are being interrupted by your baby's demands—that you are better able to cope!

9	10	11	12

WEEKS 9–12 Don't forget that your goals for each week can be anything you choose. If, up to now, showering before noon or taking a long soak in the bath one evening have seemed impossible, make that one of your weekly goals. You're not being selfish: "me time" is one of the keys to coping with this thrilling but demanding new life you have made.

MY GOALS

MONDAY

TUESDAY

WEDNESDAY

THURSDAY

FRIDAY

SATURDAY

SUNDAY

13   14   15   16

WEEKS 13–16 In pregnancy terms, the first trimester is over. How do you feel? It is a fact that regular physical activity will boost your energy levels, improve your self-image, relieve stress, and may well help you to sleep: it's a curious paradox that when you are totally exhausted attending to the needs of a small baby, you may still have trouble getting a decent night's sleep.

17 18 19 20

WEEKS 17–20 Bear in mind that, post pregnancy, your lower back and core abdominal muscles are weaker than they were before you embarked on this adventure. Your ligaments and joints also became more relaxed while you were pregnant, so it's easier to injure yourself with twisting and stretching movements. Whatever else you can't manage, don't compromise on warming up and cooling down.

MY GOALS

MONDAY

TUESDAY

WEDNESDAY

THURSDAY

FRIDAY

SATURDAY

SUNDAY

21 22 23 24

WEEKS 21–24 You're probably filling your non workout days with activities that are also contributing to your fitness levels: pushing your stroller uphill, strolling briskly around the park or to the mall, and possibly making endless trips up and down stairs. All will make a difference to how you feel and how soon your body gets back to your pre-pregnancy shape.

25 26 27 28

WEEKS 25–28 Many women want to, or find they have to, return to work around now. In terms of your baby's development it's a reasonable time: he or she is probably no longer totally reliant on your breast milk and has not yet developed an aversion to strangers. But it can make it a bit harder for you to carve out exercise time: check out if there's a gym near the office and take the cards along.

MY GOALS

MONDAY

TUESDAY

WEDNESDAY

THURSDAY

FRIDAY

SATURDAY

SUNDAY

29	30	31	32

WEEKS 29–32 Continue to pay attention to your diet: eat regular meals, drink water frequently, and avoid quick sugary fixes like chocolate and energy drinks; they contain caffeine and provide only empty calories. Snack on slow-release foods like wholegrain cereals and breads, fruit and oat-based snacks. Note what you eat and drink and how it makes you feel.

WEEKS 33–36 Take a look back on what you have achieved and how far you have come. If you feel you are losing momentum, this is a great way to motivate yourself to continue with and finish the programme. And don't be too hard on yourself: think about how far you have come from those early days when simply getting out of bed seemed an impossible achievement!

MY GOALS

MONDAY

TUESDAY

WEDNESDAY

THURSDAY

FRIDAY

SATURDAY

SUNDAY

37   38   39   40

WEEKS 37–40 Well done – you've made it! Nine months ago you completed the incredible task of bringing a new life into the world, now you've completed another milestone – getting yourself back to optimum shape and fitness. Don't stop now, however. You've laid the foundations for a lifetime of wellbeing and this needs to be maintained.

INDEX

ACKNOWLEDGMENTS

The author would like to say thank you to Jules, Chrissie, and Justine for being fun!

This book is dedicated to: my three men: Killian, Finn, and Tony

And also to my friend Karen Stevens who always reads my books and does all of the exercise routines in them!

Picture credits

Photolibrary.com
p15, p16 and p24

Food Standards Agency p15

Illustration
Amanda Williams p26

YOUR EXERCISE CARDS

On the following pages, you will find the program cards giving details of which exercises to follow and how long you need to perform them —plus a reminder to include your warm ups and cool downs. Each card contains two consecutive weeks—one to each side. Read through each exercise for the week on the core exercises pages before you start.

You now have a couple of options. You can reference your program as you would with a conventional exercise book by placing the book on the floor with the relevant card in front of you or prop it up somewhere you can see it easily as you work.

A special feature of this book, however, is that the cards are detachable for use outside the home, so that it's easy for you to take one with you if you prefer to exercise in a gym, a friend's house, or even while traveling. As you progress through the program, remove the card for the relevant week(s) and pop it in your gym bag. That way, you need only carry a single card.

When you have finished each session of your two-weekly program, you can store the card in the special pocket inside the back cover for safekeeping. You never know —you may want it again in a couple of years!

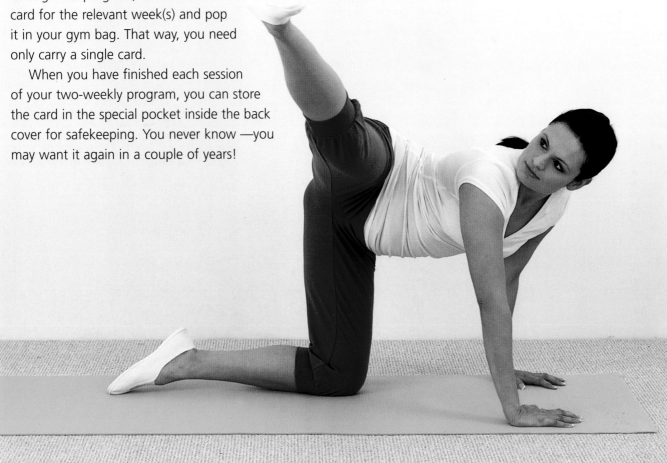

WARM UPS

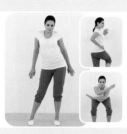

All 3 exercises, page 32
REPS: **16 of each**

PRESS UPS

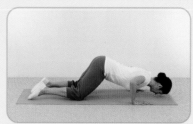

All fours position, page 63
REPS: **10**
INTENSITY: **Moderate**

STEP

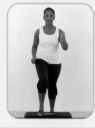

Basic step up, page 34
TIME: **3–4 minutes**
INTENSITY: **Moderate**

THIGH TONERS

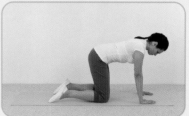

Basic all fours, page 67
REPS/TIME: **2 (hold for 20 seconds)**
INTENSITY: **Moderate**

PLANK

Basic baby plank, page 39
TIME: **20 seconds**
INTENSITY: **Moderate**

SQUATS

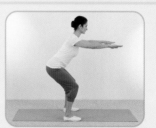

Basic squat, page 72
REPS: **10**
INTENSITY: **Light**

CURLS

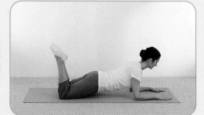

Basic curl, page 45
REPS: **5**
INTENSITY: **Moderate**

LUNGES

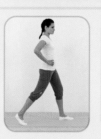

Basic lunge, page 76
REPS: **8 on each leg**
INTENSITY: **Moderate**

HYPEREXTENSION

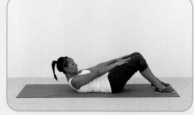

Beginner's pose, page 53
REPS: **8**
INTENSITY: **Moderate**

BODY STRETCH

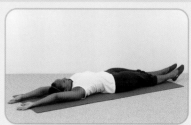

Full body stretch, page 78
REPS/TIME: **1–2 (hold for 5 seconds)**
INTENSITY: **Light**

ROLL DOWNS

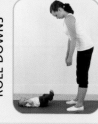 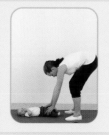

Basic roll down, page 57
REPS: **4–5 times until smooth**
INTENSITY: **Moderate**

COOL DOWNS

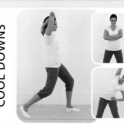

All 3 exercises, page 82
REPS/TIME: **1–2 of each (hold for 10–15 seconds with a feeling of mild tension)**

GOAL for this week...
Feel your way in, be aware of every move

WARM UPS

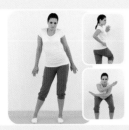

All 3 exercises, page 32
REPS: **16 of each**

STEP

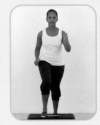

Basic step up, page 34
TIME: **3–4 minutes**
INTENSITY: **Moderate**

PLANK

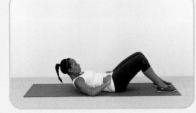

3/4 on knuckles,
page 40
TIME: **20 seconds**
INTENSITY: **Moderate**

CURLS

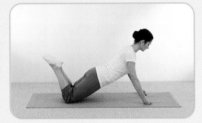

Flat curl, page 46
REPS: **8**
INTENSITY: **Moderate**

HYPEREXTENSION

Beginner's pose,
page 53
REPS: **8**
INTENSITY: **Moderate**

ROLL DOWNS

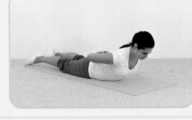

Oblique shrug, page 58
REPS: **5 on each side**
INTENSITY: **Light**

PRESS UPS

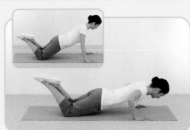

3/4 press up, page 64
REPS: **10**
INTENSITY: **Moderate**

THIGH TONERS

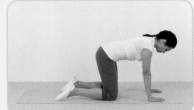

Basic all fours, page 67
REPS/TIME: **2 (hold for
20 seconds)**
INTENSITY: **Moderate**

SQUATS

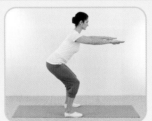

Basic squat, page 72
REPS: **10**
INTENSITY: **Light**

LUNGES

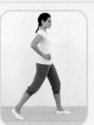 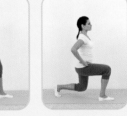

Basic lunge,
page 76
REPS: **8 on each leg**
INTENSITY: **Moderate**

BODY STRETCH

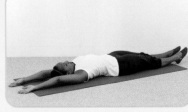

Full body stretch,
page 78
REPS/TIME: **1–2 (hold
for 5 seconds)**
INTENSITY: **Light**

COOL DOWNS

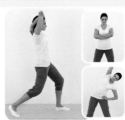

All 3 exercises, page 82
REPS/TIME: **1–2 of each (hold for
10–15 seconds with a feeling of
mild tension)**

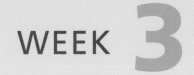

WARM UPS

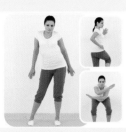

All 3 exercises, page 32
REPS: **16 of each**

PRESS UPS

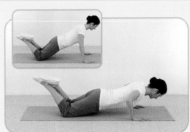

3/4 press up, page 64
REPS: **10**
INTENSITY: **Moderate**

STEP

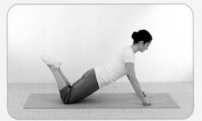

Basic step up, page 34
TIME: **3–4 minutes**
INTENSITY: **Moderate**

THIGH TONERS

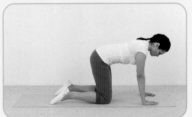

Basic all fours, page 67
REPS/TIME: **2 (hold for 20 seconds)**
INTENSITY: **Moderate**

PLANK

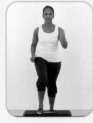

3/4 on knuckles, page 40
TIME: **20 seconds**
INTENSITY: **Moderate**

SQUATS

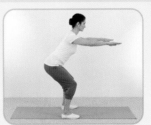

Basic squat, page 72
REPS: **10**
INTENSITY: **Light**

CURLS

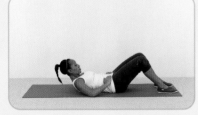

Flat curl, page 46
REPS: **8**
INTENSITY: **Moderate**

LUNGES

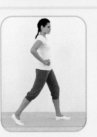

Back step lunge, page 76
REPS: **8 on each leg**
INTENSITY: **Moderate**

HYPEREXTENSION

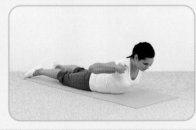

Shoulder hype, page 54
REPS: **8**
INTENSITY: **Moderate**

BODY STRETCH

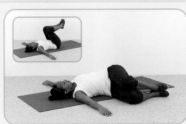

Side stretch, page 79
REPS/TIME: **1 on each side (hold for 5 seconds)**
INTENSITY: **Light**

ROLL DOWNS

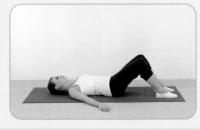

Oblique shrug, page 58
REPS: **5 on each side**
INTENSITY: **Light**

COOL DOWNS

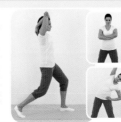

All 3 exercises, page 82
REPS/TIME: **1–2 of each (hold for 10–15 seconds with a feeling of mild tension)**

WARM UPS

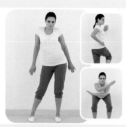
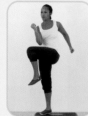
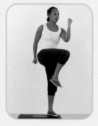

All 3 exercises, page 32
REPS: **16 of each**

PRESS UPS

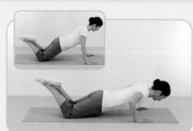

3/4 press up, page 64
REPS: **10**
INTENSITY: **Moderate**

STEP

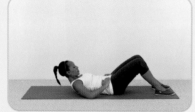

Step with knee lift, page 35
TIME: **2 minutes**
INTENSITY: **Moderate**

THIGH TONERS

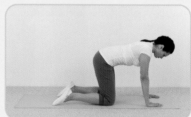

Basic all fours, page 67
REPS/TIME: **2 (hold for 20 seconds)**
INTENSITY: **Moderate**

PLANK

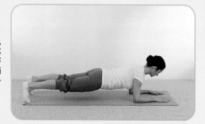

Full plank, page 40
TIME: **20 seconds**
INTENSITY: **Moderate**

SQUATS

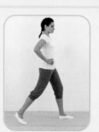
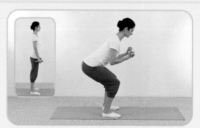

Squat with bicep curl, page 73
REPS: **10**
INTENSITY: **Light**

CURLS

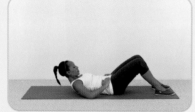

Flat curl, page 46
REPS: **8**
INTENSITY: **Moderate**

LUNGES

Back step lunge, page 76
REPS: **8 on each leg**
INTENSITY: **Moderate**

HYPEREXTENSION

Shoulder hype, page 54
REPS: **8**
INTENSITY: **Moderate**

BODY STRETCH

Side stretch, page 79
REPS/TIME: **1 on each side (hold for 5 seconds)**
INTENSITY: **Light**

ROLL DOWNS

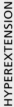
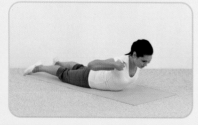

Hip hitch, page 58
REPS: **8 on each side**
INTENSITY: **Light**

COOL DOWNS

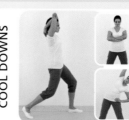
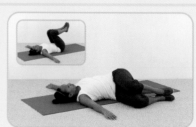
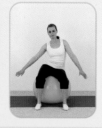
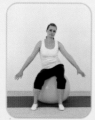

All 3 exercises, page 82
REPS/TIME: **1–2 of each (hold for 10–15 seconds with a feeling of mild tension)**

GOAL for this week...
Now you're into it, keep it going

WARM UPS

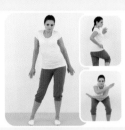

All 3 exercises, page 32
REPS: **16 of each**

PRESS UPS

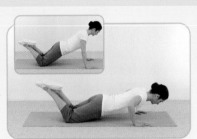

3/4 press up, page 64
REPS: **10**
INTENSITY: **Moderate**

STEP

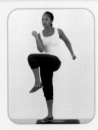
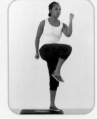

Step with knee lift, page 35
TIME: **2 minutes**
INTENSITY: **Moderate**

THIGH TONERS

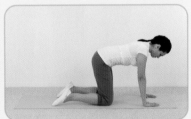

Basic all fours, page 67
REPS/TIME: **2 (hold for 20 seconds)**
INTENSITY: **Moderate**

PLANK

Full plank, page 40
TIME: **20 seconds**
INTENSITY: **Moderate**

SQUATS

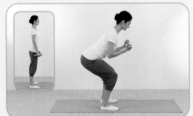

Squat with bicep curl, page 73
REPS: **10**
INTENSITY: **Light**

CURLS

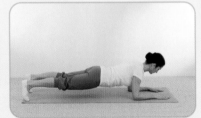

Flat curl, page 46
REPS: **8**
INTENSITY: **Moderate**

LUNGES

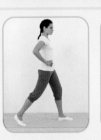

Back step lunge, page 76
REPS: **8 on each leg**
INTENSITY: **Moderate**

HYPEREXTENSION

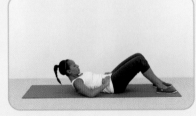

Shoulder hype, page 54
REPS: **8**
INTENSITY: **Moderate**

BODY STRETCH

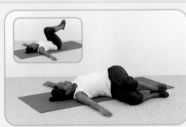

Side stretch, page 79
REPS/TIME: **1 on each side (hold for 5 seconds)**
INTENSITY: **Light**

ROLL DOWNS

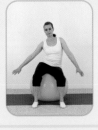
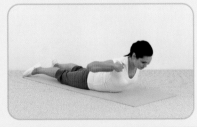

Hip hitch, page 58
REPS: **8 on each side**
INTENSITY: **Light**

COOL DOWNS

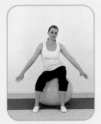

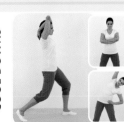

All 3 exercises, page 82
REPS/TIME: **1–2 of each (hold for 10–15 seconds with a feeling of mild tension)**

GOAL for this week...
Really begin to reconnect to your abdominals

WARM UPS

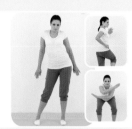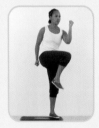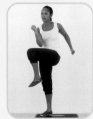

All 3 exercises, page 32
REPS: **16 of each**

PRESS UPS

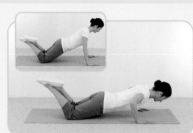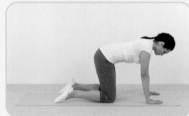

3/4 press up, page 64
REPS: **10**
INTENSITY: **Moderate**

STEP

Step with knee lift, page 35
TIME: **2 minutes**
INTENSITY: **Moderate**

THIGH TONERS

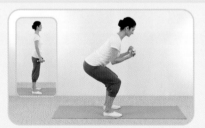

Basic all fours, page 67
REPS/TIME: **2 (hold for 20 seconds)**
INTENSITY: **Moderate**

PLANK

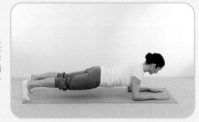

Full plank, page 40
TIME: **20 seconds**
INTENSITY: **Moderate**

SQUATS

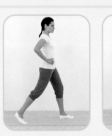

Squat with bicep curl, page 73
REPS: **10**
INTENSITY: **Light**

CURLS

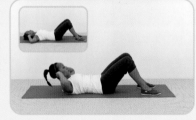

Full curl, page 46
REPS: **10**
INTENSITY: **Moderate**

LUNGES

Back step lunge, page 76
REPS: **8 on each leg**
INTENSITY: **Moderate**

HYPEREXTENSION

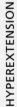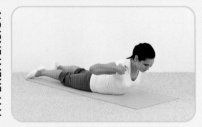

Shoulder hype, page 54
REPS: **8**
INTENSITY: **Moderate**

BODY STRETCH

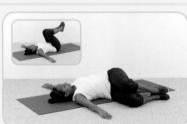

Side stretch, page 79
REPS/TIME: **1 on each side (hold for 5 seconds)**
INTENSITY: **Light**

ROLL DOWNS

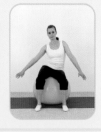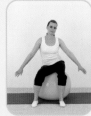

Hip hitch, page 58
REPS: **8 on each side**
INTENSITY: **Light**

COOL DOWNS

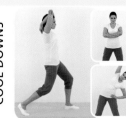

All 3 exercises, page 82
REPS/TIME: **1–2 of each (hold for 10–15 seconds with a feeling of mild tension)**

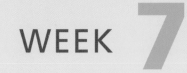
WARM UPS

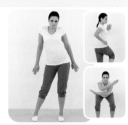

All 3 exercises, page 32
REPS: **16 of each**

PRESS UPS

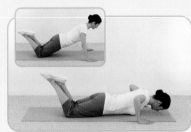

Wide arm press up,
page 64
REPS: **10**
INTENSITY: **Moderate**

STEP

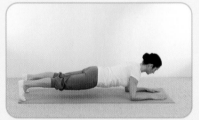

Step with knee lift,
page 35
TIME: **2 minutes**
INTENSITY: **Moderate**

THIGH TONERS

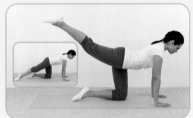

Back kick, page 68
REPS: **10 on each leg**
INTENSITY: **Moderate**

PLANK

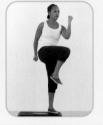

Full plank, page 40
TIME: **20 seconds**
INTENSITY: **Moderate**

SQUATS

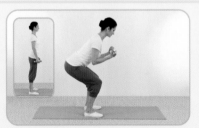

Squat with bicep curl,
page 73
REPS: **10**
INTENSITY: **Light**

CURLS

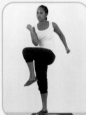

Full curl, page 46
REPS: **10**
INTENSITY: **Moderate**

LUNGES

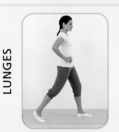

Back step lunge,
page 76
REPS: **8 on each leg**
INTENSITY: **Moderate**

HYPEREXTENSION

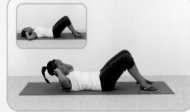

Shoulder hype,
page 54
REPS: **8**
INTENSITY: **Moderate**

BODY STRETCH

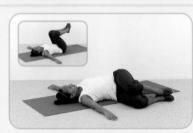

Side stretch, page 79
REPS/TIME: **1 on each
side (hold for
5 seconds)**
INTENSITY: **Light**

ROLL DOWNS

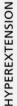 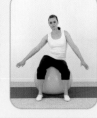 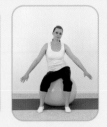

Hip hitch, page 58
REPS: **8 on each side**
INTENSITY: **Light**

COOL DOWNS

 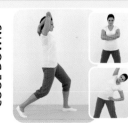

All 3 exercises, page 82
REPS/TIME: **1–2 of each (hold for
10–15 seconds with a feeling of
mild tension)**

WARM UPS

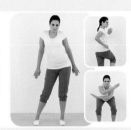 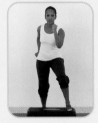 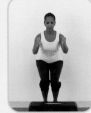

All 3 exercises, page 32
REPS: **16 of each**

PRESS UPS

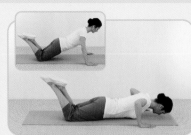

Wide arm press up, page 64
REPS: **10**
INTENSITY: **Moderate**

STEP

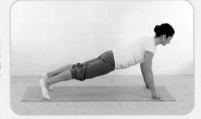

Step with squats, page 36
TIME: **2 minutes**
INTENSITY: **Moderate**

THIGH TONERS

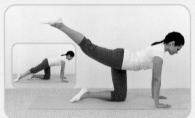

Back kick, page 68
REPS: **10 on each leg**
INTENSITY: **Moderate**

PLANK

Full plank on knuckles, page 40
TIME: **30 seconds**
INTENSITY: **Vigorous**

SQUATS

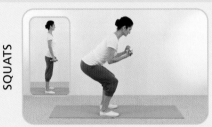

Squat with bicep curl, page 73
REPS: **10**
INTENSITY: **Light**

CURLS

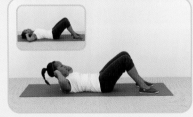

Full curl, page 46
REPS: **10**
INTENSITY: **Moderate**

LUNGES

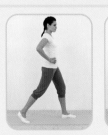

Back step lunge, page 76
REPS: **8 on each leg**
INTENSITY: **Moderate**

HYPEREXTENSION

Shoulder hype, page 54
REPS: **8**
INTENSITY: **Moderate**

BODY STRETCH

Side stretch, page 79
REPS/TIME: **1 on each side (hold for 5 seconds)**
INTENSITY: **Light**

ROLL DOWNS

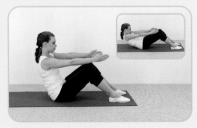

Straight arm roll down, page 59
REPS: **3–4**
INTENSITY: **Moderate**

COOL DOWNS

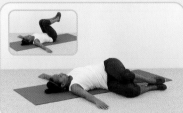 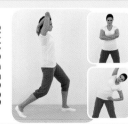 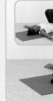

All 3 exercises, page 82
REPS/TIME: **1–2 of each (hold for 10–15 seconds with a feeling of mild tension)**

WARM UPS

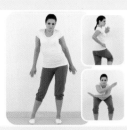 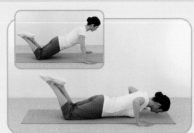

All 3 exercises, page 32
REPS: **16 of each**

PRESS UPS

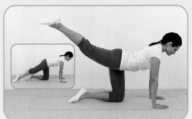

Wide arm press up, page 64
REPS: **10**
INTENSITY: **Moderate**

STEP

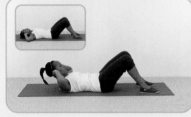

Step with squats, page 36
TIME: **2 minutes**
INTENSITY: **Moderate**

THIGH TONERS

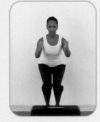 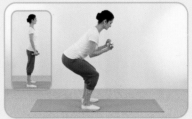

Back kick, page 68
REPS: **10 on each leg**
INTENSITY: **Moderate**

PLANK

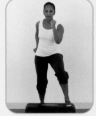 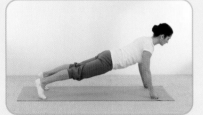

Full plank on knuckles, page 40
TIME: **30 seconds**
INTENSITY: **Vigorous**

SQUATS

 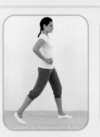

Squat with bicep curl, page 73
REPS: **10**
INTENSITY: **Light**

CURLS

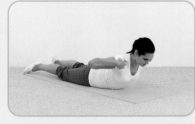

Full curl, page 46
REPS: **10**
INTENSITY: **Moderate**

LUNGES

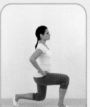 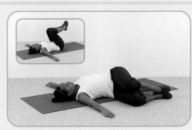

Back step lunge, page 76
REPS: **8 on each leg**
INTENSITY: **Moderate**

HYPEREXTENSION

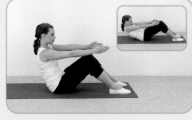

Shoulder hype, page 54
REPS: **8**
INTENSITY: **Moderate**

BODY STRETCH

Side stretch, page 79
REPS/TIME: **1 on each side (hold for 5 seconds)**
INTENSITY: **Light**

ROLL DOWNS

Straight arm roll down, page 59
REPS: **3–4**
INTENSITY: **Moderate**

COOL DOWNS

 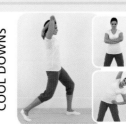

All 3 exercises, page 82
REPS/TIME: **1–2 of each (hold for 10–15 seconds with a feeling of mild tension)**

GOAL for this week...
Master the ball!

WARM UPS

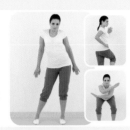 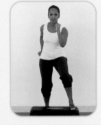 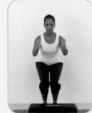

All 3 exercises, page 32
REPS: **16 of each**

PRESS UPS

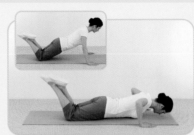

Wide arm press up,
page 64
REPS: **10**
INTENSITY: **Moderate**

STEP

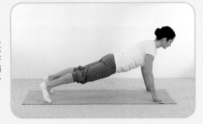

Step with squats,
page 36
TIME: **2 minutes**
INTENSITY: **Moderate**

THIGH TONERS

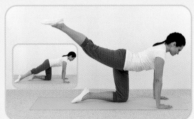

Back kick, page 68
REPS: **10 on each leg**
INTENSITY: **Moderate**

PLANK

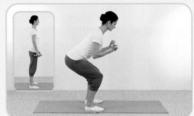

Full plank on knuckles,
page 40
TIME: **30 seconds**
INTENSITY: **Vigorous**

SQUATS

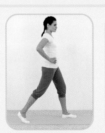

Squat with bicep curl,
page 73
REPS: **10**
INTENSITY: **Light**

CURLS

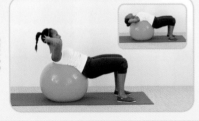

Ball ab curl, page 47
REPS: **15**
INTENSITY: **Moderate**

LUNGES

Back step lunge,
page 76
REPS: **8 on each leg**
INTENSITY: **Moderate**

HYPEREXTENSION

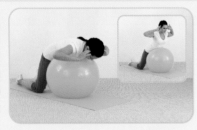

Ball arch, page 54
REPS: **10**
INTENSITY: **Moderate**

BODY STRETCH

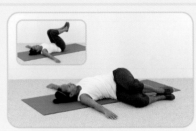

Side stretch, page 79
REPS/TIME: **1 on each
side** (hold for
5 seconds)
INTENSITY: **Light**

ROLL DOWNS

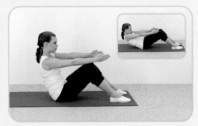

Straight arm roll
down, page 59
REPS: **3–4**
INTENSITY: **Moderate**

COOL DOWNS

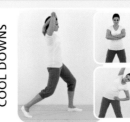

All 3 exercises, page 82
REPS/TIME: **1–2 of each** (hold for
10–15 seconds with a feeling of
mild tension)

GOAL for this week...
Get your roll downs working really smoothly

WARM UPS
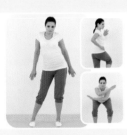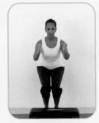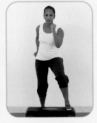
All 3 exercises, page 32
REPS: **16 of each**

STEP
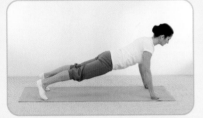
Step with squats, page 36
TIME: **2 minutes**
INTENSITY: **Moderate**

PLANK
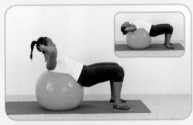
Full plank on knuckles, page 40
TIME: **30 seconds**
INTENSITY: **Vigorous**

CURLS

Ball ab curl, page 47
REPS: **15**
INTENSITY: **Moderate**

HYPEREXTENSION
Ball arch, page 54
REPS: **10**
INTENSITY: **Moderate**

ROLL DOWNS
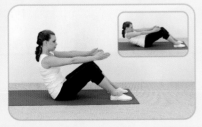
Straight arm roll down, page 59
REPS: **3–4**
INTENSITY: **Moderate**

PRESS UPS
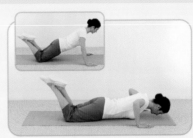
Wide arm press up, page 64
REPS: **10**
INTENSITY: **Moderate**

THIGH TONERS
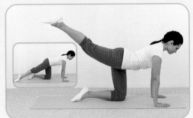
Back kick, page 68
REPS: **10 on each leg**
INTENSITY: **Moderate**

SQUATS
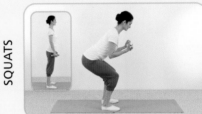
Squat with bicep curl, page 73
REPS: **10**
INTENSITY: **Light**

LUNGES
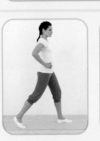
Back step lunge, page 76
REPS: **8 on each leg**
INTENSITY: **Moderate**

BODY STRETCH
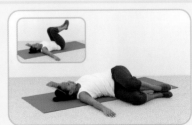
Side stretch, page 79
REPS/TIME: **1 on each side (hold for 5 seconds)**
INTENSITY: **Light**

COOL DOWNS
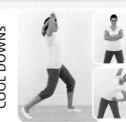
All 3 exercises, page 82
REPS/TIME: **1–2 of each (hold for 10–15 seconds with a feeling of mild tension)**

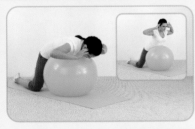

GOAL for this week... Go for higher kicks on the step (as long as you're warm!)

WARM UPS

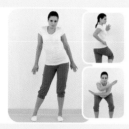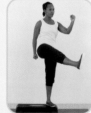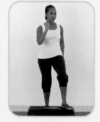

All 3 exercises, page 32
REPS: **16 of each**

STEP

Step with kick, page 36
TIME: **2 minutes**
INTENSITY: **Moderate**

PLANK

Foot lift, page 41
TIME: **30 seconds (with lifting and lowering)**
INTENSITY: **Vigorous**

CURLS

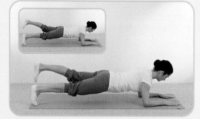

Ball ab curl, page 47
REPS: **15**
INTENSITY: **Moderate**

HYPEREXTENSION

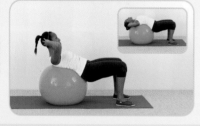

Ball arch, page 54
REPS: **10**
INTENSITY: **Moderate**

ROLL DOWNS

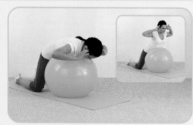

Straight arm roll down, page 59
REPS: **3–4**
INTENSITY: **Moderate**

PRESS UPS

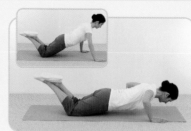

Uneven arm press, page 65
REPS: **10 with each hand in front**
INTENSITY: **Moderate**

THIGH TONERS

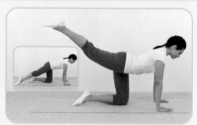

Back kick, page 68
REPS: **10 on each leg**
INTENSITY: **Moderate**

SQUATS

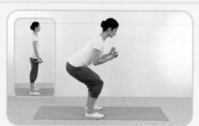

Squat with bicep curl, page 73
REPS: **10**
INTENSITY: **Light**

LUNGES

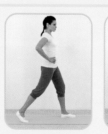

Back step lunge, page 76
REPS: **8 on each leg**
INTENSITY: **Moderate**

BODY STRETCH

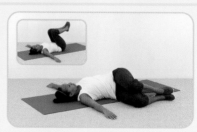

Side stretch, page 79
REPS/TIME: **1 on each side (hold for 5 seconds)**
INTENSITY: **Light**

COOL DOWNS

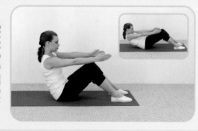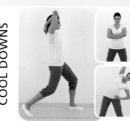

All 3 exercises, page 82
REPS/TIME: **1–2 of each (hold for 10–15 seconds with a feeling of mild tension)**

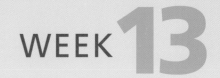
WARM UPS

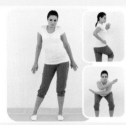

All 3 exercises, page 32
REPS: **16 of each**

STEP

**Step with kick,
page 36**
TIME: **2 minutes**
INTENSITY: **Moderate**

PLANK

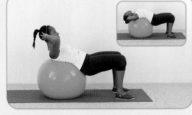

Foot lift, page 41
TIME: **30 seconds (with
lifting and lowering)**
INTENSITY: **Vigorous**

CURLS

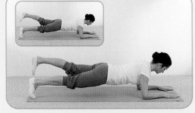

Ball ab curl, page 47
REPS: **15**
INTENSITY: **Moderate**

HYPEREXTENSION

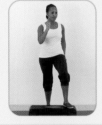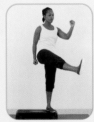

Ball arch, page 54
REPS: **10**
INTENSITY: **Moderate**

ROLL DOWNS

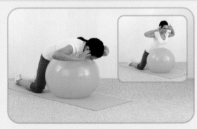

**Cross your heart roll
down, page 60**
REPS: **3–4**
INTENSITY: **Moderate**

PRESS UPS

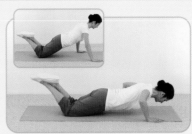

**Uneven arm press,
page 65**
REPS: **10 with each
hand in front**
INTENSITY: **Moderate**

THIGH TONERS

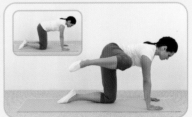

Donkey lift, page 68
REPS: **10 on each leg**
INTENSITY: **Moderate**

SQUATS

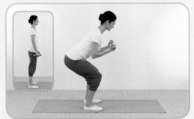

**Squat with bicep curl,
page 73**
REPS: **10**
INTENSITY: **Light**

LUNGES

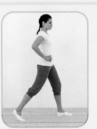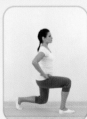

**Back step lunge,
page 76**
REPS: **8 on each leg**
INTENSITY: **Moderate**

BODY STRETCH

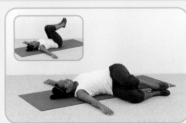

Side stretch, page 79
REPS/TIME: **1 on each
side (hold for
5 seconds)**
INTENSITY: **Light**

COOL DOWNS

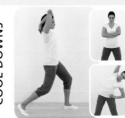

All 3 exercises, page 82
REPS/TIME: **1–2 of each (hold for
10–15 seconds with a feeling of
mild tension)**

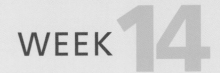

GOAL for this week...
Keep your buttock muscles tightened throughout

WARM UPS

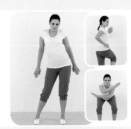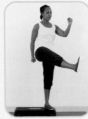

All 3 exercises, page 32
REPS: **16 of each**

STEP

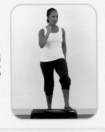

Step with kick, page 36
TIME: **2 minutes**
INTENSITY: **Moderate**

PLANK

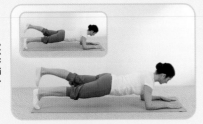

Foot lift, page 41
TIME: **30 seconds (with lifting and lowering)**
INTENSITY: **Vigorous**

CURLS

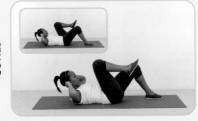

Knee curl, page 48
REPS: **15 on each alternating leg**
INTENSITY: **Moderate**

HYPEREXTENSION

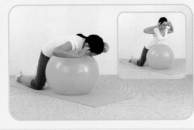

Ball arch, page 54
REPS: **10**
INTENSITY: **Moderate**

ROLL DOWNS

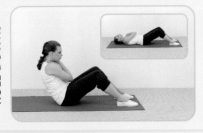

Cross your heart roll down, page 60
REPS: **3–4**
INTENSITY: **Moderate**

PRESS UPS

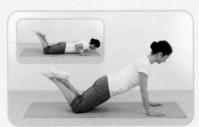

Tri press, page 65
REPS: **15**
INTENSITY: **Moderate**

THIGH TONERS

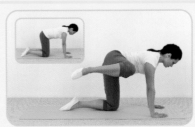

Donkey lift, page 68
REPS: **10 on each leg**
INTENSITY: **Moderate**

SQUATS

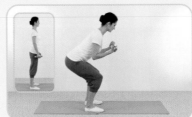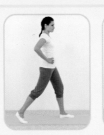

Squat with bicep curl, page 73
REPS: **10**
INTENSITY: **Light**

LUNGES

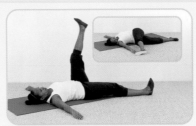

Back step lunge, page 76
REPS: **8 on each leg**
INTENSITY: **Moderate**

BODY STRETCH

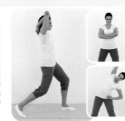

Raised leg stretch, page 80
REPS/TIME: **1 on each side (hold for 10 seconds)**
INTENSITY: **Light**

COOL DOWNS

All 3 exercises, page 82
REPS/TIME: **1–2 of each (hold for 10–15 seconds with a feeling of mild tension)**

WARM UPS

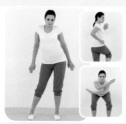
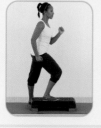

All 3 exercises, page 32
REPS: **16 of each**

STEP

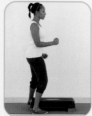

Sideways, page 37
TIME: **2 minutes**
INTENSITY: **Moderate**

PLANK

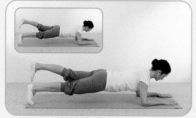

Foot lift, page 41
TIME: **30 seconds (with lifting and lowering)**
INTENSITY: **Vigorous**

CURLS

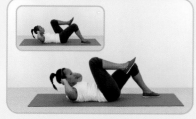

Knee curl, page 48
REPS: **15 on each alternating leg**
INTENSITY: **Moderate**

HYPEREXTENSION

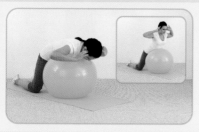

Ball arch, page 54
REPS: **10**
INTENSITY: **Moderate**

ROLL DOWNS

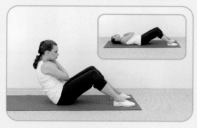

Cross your heart roll down, page 60
REPS: **3–4**
INTENSITY: **Moderate**

PRESS-UPS

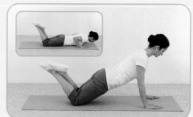

Tri press, page 65
REPS: **15**
INTENSITY: **Moderate**

THIGH TONERS

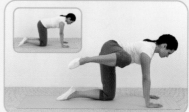

Donkey lift, page 68
REPS: **10 on each leg**
INTENSITY: **Moderate**

SQUATS

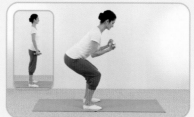

Squat with bicep curl, page 73
REPS: **10**
INTENSITY: **Light**

LUNGES

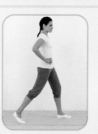

Back step lunge, page 76
REPS: **8 on each leg**
INTENSITY: **Moderate**

BODY STRETCH

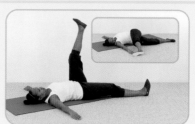

Raised leg stretch, page 80
REPS/TIME: **1 on each side (hold for 10 seconds)**
INTENSITY: **Light**

COOL DOWNS

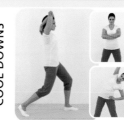

All 3 exercises, page 82
REPS/TIME: **1–2 of each (hold for 10–15 seconds with a feeling of mild tension)**

GOAL for this week... Concentrate on breathing regularly throughout every exercise

WEEK **16**

WARM UPS

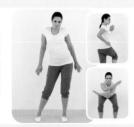

All 3 exercises, page 32
REPS: **16 of each**

STEP

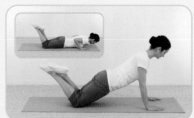

Sideways, page 37
TIME: **2 minutes**
INTENSITY: **Moderate**

PLANK

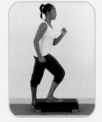

Step it, page 41
TIME: **30 seconds**
(while moving feet)
INTENSITY: **Vigorous**

CURLS

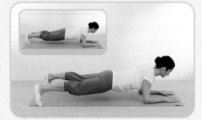

Knee curl, page 48
REPS: **15 on each**
alternating leg
INTENSITY: **Moderate**

HYPEREXTENSION

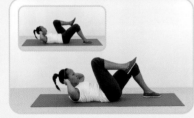

Ball arch, page 54
REPS: **10**
INTENSITY: **Moderate**

ROLL DOWNS

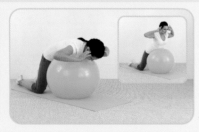

Shoulder shrug roll,
page 60
REPS: **3–4**
INTENSITY: **Moderate**

PRESS UPS

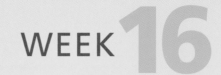

Tri press, page 65
REPS: **15**
INTENSITY: **Moderate**

THIGH TONERS

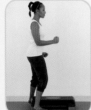

Donkey lift, page 68
REPS: **10 on each leg**
INTENSITY: **Moderate**

SQUATS

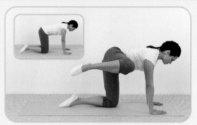

Squat with bicep curl,
page 73
REPS: **10**
INTENSITY: **Light**

LUNGES

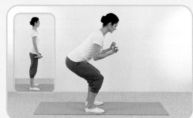

Back step lunge,
page 76
REPS: **8 on each leg**
INTENSITY: **Moderate**

BODY STRETCH

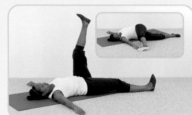

Raised leg stretch,
page 80
REPS/TIME:**1 on each**
side (hold for
10 seconds)
INTENSITY: **Light**

COOL DOWNS

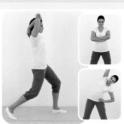 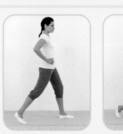 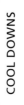 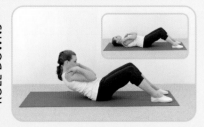

All 3 exercises, page 82
REPS/TIME: **1–2 of each (hold for**
10–15 seconds with a feeling of
mild tension)

GOAL for this week... Stretch out your spine to lift higher on back extensions

WARM UPS

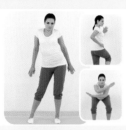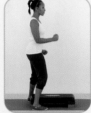

All 3 exercises, page 32
REPS: **16 of each**

PRESS UPS

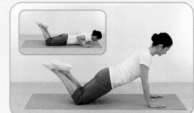

Tri press, page 65
REPS: **15**
INTENSITY: **Moderate**

STEP

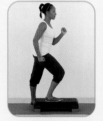

Sideways, page 37
TIME: **2 minutes**
INTENSITY: **Moderate**

THIGH TONERS

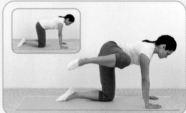

Donkey lift, page 68
REPS: **10 on each leg**
INTENSITY: **Moderate**

PLANK

Step it, page 41
TIME: **30 seconds
(while moving feet)**
INTENSITY: **Vigorous**

SQUATS

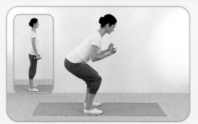

**Squat with bicep curl,
page 73**
REPS: **10**
INTENSITY: **Light**

CURLS

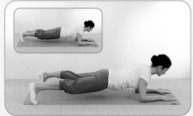

Knee curl, page 48
REPS: **15 on each
alternating leg**
INTENSITY: **Moderate**

LUNGES

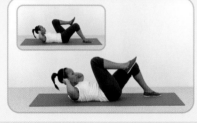

**Back step lunge,
page 76**
REPS: **8 on each leg**
INTENSITY: **Moderate**

HYPEREXTENSION

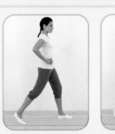

**Straight arm ball arch,
page 55**
REPS: **12**
INTENSITY: **Moderate**

BODY STRETCH

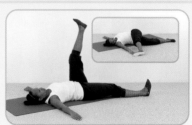

**Raised leg stretch,
page 80**
REPS/TIME: **1 on each
side (hold for
10 seconds)**
INTENSITY: **Light**

ROLL DOWNS

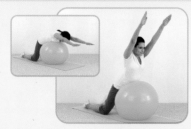

**Shoulder shrug roll,
page 60**
REPS: **3–4**
INTENSITY: **Moderate**

COOL DOWNS

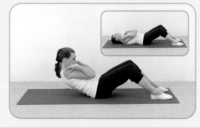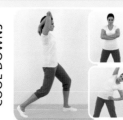

All 3 exercises, page 82
REPS/TIME: **1–2 of each (hold for
10–15 seconds with a feeling of
mild tension)**

WARM UPS

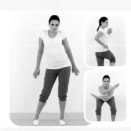

All 3 exercises, page 32
REPS: **16 of each**

PRESS UPS

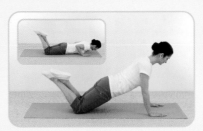

Tri press, page 65
REPS: **15**
INTENSITY: **Moderate**

STEP

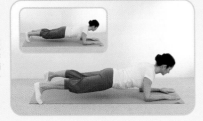

Sideways, page 37
TIME: **2 minutes**
INTENSITY: **Moderate**

THIGH TONER

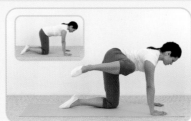

Donkey lift, page 68
REPS: **10 on each leg**
INTENSITY: **Moderate**

PLANK

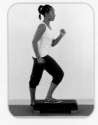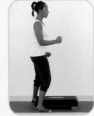

Step it, page 41
TIME: **30 seconds**
(while moving feet)
INTENSITY: **Vigorous**

SQUATS

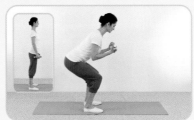

**Squat with bicep curl,
page 73**
REPS: **10**
INTENSITY: **Light**

CURLS

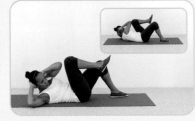

Diagonal curl, page 49
REPS: **15 on each
alternating leg**
INTENSITY: **Moderate**

LUNGES

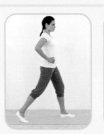

**Back step lunge,
page 76**
REPS: **8 on each leg**
INTENSITY: **Moderate**

HYPEREXTENSION

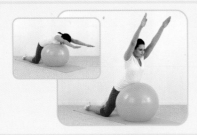

**Straight arm ball arch,
page 55**
REPS: **12**
INTENSITY: **Moderate**

BODY STRETCH

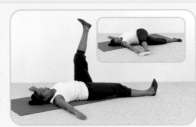

**Raised leg stretch,
page 80**
REPS/TIME: **1 on each
side (hold for
10 seconds)**
INTENSITY: **Light**

ROLL DOWNS

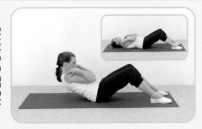

**Shoulder shrug roll,
page 60**
REPS: **3–4**
INTENSITY: **Moderate**

COOL DOWNS

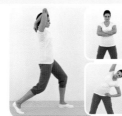

All 3 exercises, page 82
REPS/TIME: **1–2 of each (hold for
10–15 seconds with a feeling of
mild tension)**

GOAL for this week... Aim to keep your weight on your heels in the squat move

WARM UPS

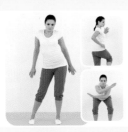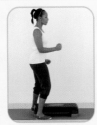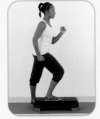

All 3 exercises, page 32
REPS: **16 of each**

PRESS UPS

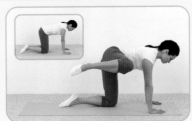

Tri press, page 65
REPS: **15**
INTENSITY: **Moderate**

STEP

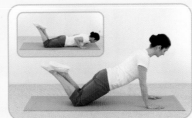

Sideways, page 37
TIME: **2 minutes**
INTENSITY: **Moderate**

THIGH TONERS

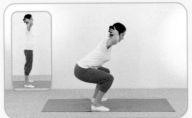

Donkey lift, page 68
REPS: **10 on each leg**
INTENSITY: **Moderate**

PLANK

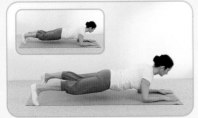

Step it, page 41
TIME: **30 seconds
(while moving feet)**
INTENSITY: **Vigorous**

SQUATS

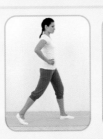

Prisoner squat,
page 73
REPS: **10**
INTENSITY: **Moderate**

CURLS

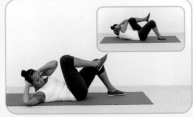

Diagonal curl, page 49
REPS: **15 on each
alternating leg**
INTENSITY: **Moderate**

LUNGES

Back step lunge,
page 76
REPS: **8 on each leg**
INTENSITY: **Moderate**

HYPEREXTENSION

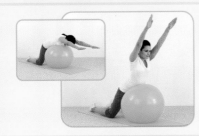

Straight arm ball arch,
page 55
REPS: **12**
INTENSITY: **Moderate**

BODY STRETCH

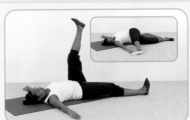

Raised leg stretch,
page 80
REPS/TIME:**1 on each
side (hold for
10 seconds)**
INTENSITY: **Light**

ROLL DOWNS

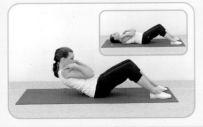

Shoulder shrug roll,
page 60
REPS: **3–4**
INTENSITY: **Moderate**

COOL DOWNS

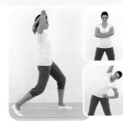

All 3 exercises, page 82
REPS/TIME: **1–2 of each (hold for
10–15 seconds with a feeling of
mild tension)**

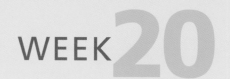

GOAL for this week... Keep your hips and stomach well lifted in the plank move

WARM UPS

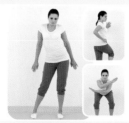
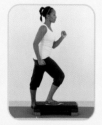
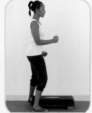

All 3 exercises, page 32
REPS: **16 of each**

STEP

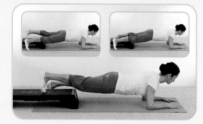

Sideways, page 37
TIME: **2 minutes**
INTENSITY: **Moderate**

PLANK

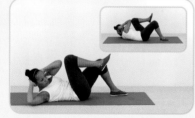

Step ups, page 42
TIME: **30 seconds
(while moving feet)**
INTENSITY: **Vigorous**

CURLS

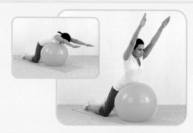

Diagonal curl, page 49
REPS: **15 on each
alternating leg**
INTENSITY: **Moderate**

HYPEREXTENSION

Straight arm ball arch,
page 55
REPS: **12**
INTENSITY: **Moderate**

ROLL DOWNS

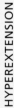
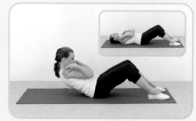

Shoulder shrug roll,
page 60
REPS: **3–4**
INTENSITY: **Moderate**

PRESS UPS

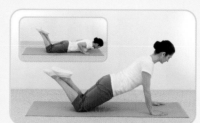

Tri press, page 65
REPS: **15**
INTENSITY: **Moderate**

THIGH TONERS

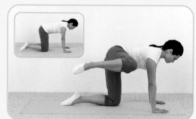

Donkey lift, page 68
REPS: **10 on each leg**
INTENSITY: **Moderate**

SQUATS

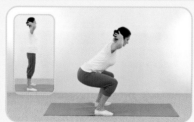

Prisoner squat,
page 73
REPS: **10**
INTENSITY: **Moderate**

LUNGES

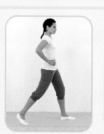

Back step lunge,
page 76
REPS: **8 on each leg**
INTENSITY: **Moderate**

BODY STRETCH

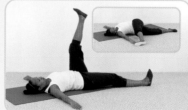

Raised leg stretch,
page 80
REPS/TIME:**1 on each
side (hold for
10 seconds)**
INTENSITY: **Light**

COOL DOWNS

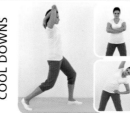

All 3 exercises, page 82
REPS/TIME: **1–2 of each (hold for
10–15 seconds with a feeling of
mild tension)**

GOAL for this week...
Really control the curl motion in your roll downs

WARM UPS

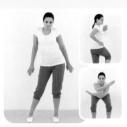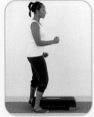

All 3 exercises, page 32
REPS: **16 of each**

PRESS UPS

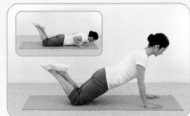

Tri press, page 65
REPS: **15**
INTENSITY: **Moderate**

STEP

All 3 exercises, page 32

Sideways, page 37
TIME: **2 minutes**
INTENSITY: **Moderate**

THIGH TONERS

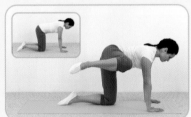

Donkey lift, page 68
REPS: **10 on each leg**
INTENSITY: **Moderate**

PLANK

Step ups, page 42
TIME: **30 seconds while moving feet**
INTENSITY: **Vigorous**

SQUATS

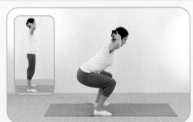

Prisoner squat, page 73
REPS: **10**
INTENSITY: **Moderate**

CURLS

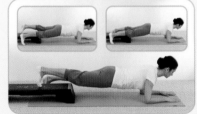

Diagonal curl, page 49
REPS: **15 on each alternating leg**
INTENSITY: **Moderate**

LUNGES

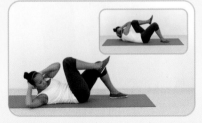

Back step lunge, page 76
REPS: **8 on each leg**
INTENSITY: **Moderate**

HYPEREXTENSION

Straight arm ball arch, page 55
REPS: **12**
INTENSITY: **Moderate**

BODY STRETCH

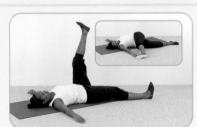

Raised leg stretch, page 80
REPS/TIME: **1 on each side (hold for 10 seconds)**
INTENSITY: **Light**

ROLL DOWNS

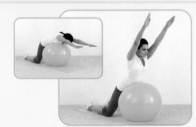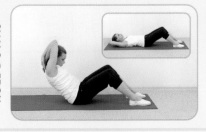

Necklace roll down, page 61
REPS: **3–4**
INTENSITY: **Moderate**

COOL DOWNS

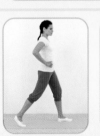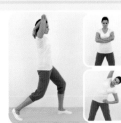

All 3 exercises, page 82
REPS/TIME: **1–2 of each (hold for 10–15 seconds with a feeling of mild tension)**

GOAL for this week...
Jump up high on the step

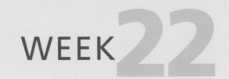

WARM UPS
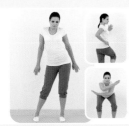
All 3 exercises, page 32
REPS: 16 of each

STEP
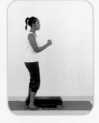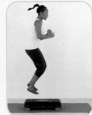
With jumps, page 37
REPS: 10
INTENSITY: Vigorous

PLANK
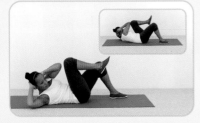
Step ups, page 42
TIME: 30 seconds while moving feet
INTENSITY: Vigorous

CURLS
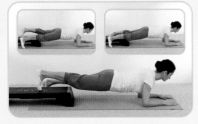
Diagonal curl, page 49
REPS: 15 on each alternating leg
INTENSITY: Moderate

HYPEREXTENSION
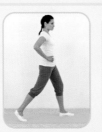
Straight arm ball arch, page 55
REPS: 12
INTENSITY: Moderate

ROLL DOWNS
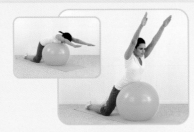
Necklace roll down, page 61
REPS: 3–4
INTENSITY: Moderate

PRESS UPS
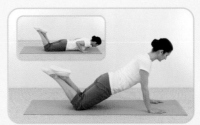
Tri press, page 65
REPS: 15
INTENSITY: Moderate

THIGH TONERS
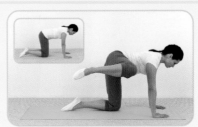
Donkey lift, page 68
REPS: 10 on each leg
INTENSITY: Moderate

SQUATS
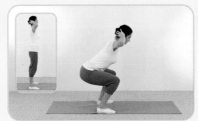
Prisoner squat, page 73
REPS: 10
INTENSITY: Moderate

LUNGES
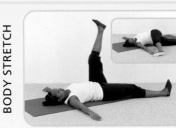
Back step lunge, page 76
REPS: 8 on each leg
INTENSITY: Moderate

BODY STRETCH
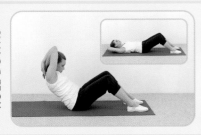
Raised leg stretch, page 80
REPS/TIME: 1 on each side (hold for 10 seconds)
INTENSITY: Light

COOL DOWNS
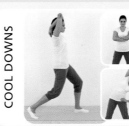
All 3 exercises, page 82
REPS/TIME: 1–2 of each (hold for 10–15 seconds with a feeling of mild tension)

GOAL for this week... Take extra care to keep your hips, knees, and toes aligned as you bend your knees

WARM UPS

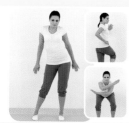

All 3 exercises, page 32
REPS: **16 of each**

STEP

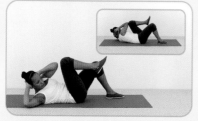

With jumps, page 37
REPS: **10**
INTENSITY: **Vigorous**

PLANK

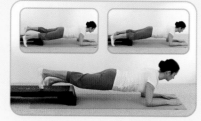

Step ups, page 42
TIME: **30 seconds while moving feet**
INTENSITY: **Vigorous**

CURLS

Diagonal curl, page 49
REPS: **15 on each alternating leg**
INTENSITY: **Moderate**

HYPEREXTENSION

Straight arm ball arch, page 55
REPS: **12**
INTENSITY: **Moderate**

ROLL DOWNS

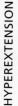
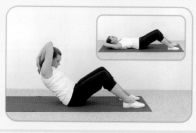

Necklace roll down, page 61
REPS: **3–4**
INTENSITY: **Moderate**

PRESS UPS

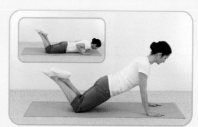

Tri press, page 65
REPS: **15**
INTENSITY: **Moderate**

THIGH TONERS

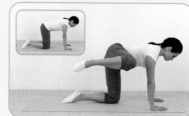

Donkey lift, page 68
REPS: **10 on each leg**
INTENSITY: **Moderate**

SQUATS

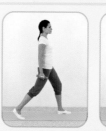

Prisoner squat, page 73
REPS: **10**
INTENSITY: **Moderate**

LUNGES

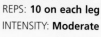
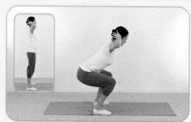

Forward step lunge, page 77
REPS: **10 on each leg**
INTENSITY: **Moderate**

BODY STRETCH

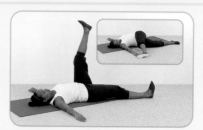

Raised leg stretch, page 80
REPS/TIME: **1 on each side (hold for 10 seconds)**
INTENSITY: **Light**

COOL DOWNS

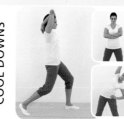

All 3 exercises, page 82
REPS/TIME: **1–2 of each (hold for 10–15 seconds with a feeling of mild tension)**

GOAL for this week... Focus on getting a range of movement – go as low as possible with every move

WARM UPS

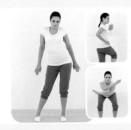

All 3 exercises, page 32
REPS: **16 of each**

STEP

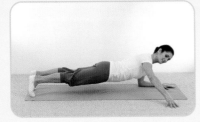

With jumps, page 37
REPS: **10**
INTENSITY: **Vigorous**

PLANK

Touch line, page 42
TIME: **30 seconds while moving arms**
INTENSITY: **Vigorous**

CURLS

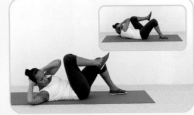

Diagonal curl, page 49
REPS: **15 on each alternating leg**
INTENSITY: **Moderate**

HYPEREXTENSION

Leg fly, page 55
REPS: **8**
INTENSITY: **Moderate**

ROLL DOWNS

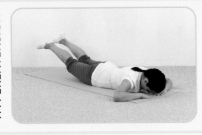

Necklace roll down, page 61
REPS: **3–4**
INTENSITY: **Moderate**

PRESS UPS

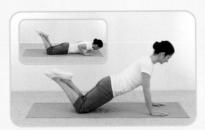

Tri press, page 65
REPS: **15**
INTENSITY: **Moderate**

THIGH TONERS

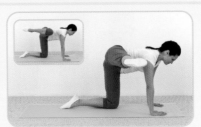

Donkey kick, page 69
REPS: **10 on each leg**
INTENSITY: **Moderate**

SQUATS

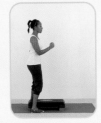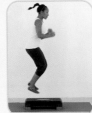

Prisoner squat, page 73
REPS: **10**
INTENSITY: **Moderate**

LUNGES

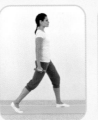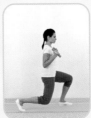

Forward step lunge, page 77
REPS: **10 on each leg**
INTENSITY: **Moderate**

BODY STRETCH

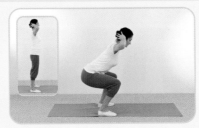

Raised leg stretch, page 80
REPS/TIME: **1 on each side (hold for 10 seconds)**
INTENSITY: **Light**

COOL DOWNS

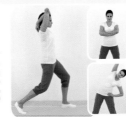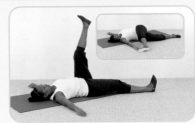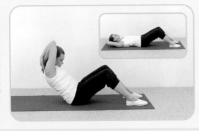

All 3 exercises, page 82
REPS/TIME: **1–2 of each (hold for 10-15 seconds with a feeling of mild tension)**

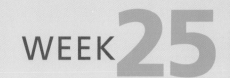

WARM UPS

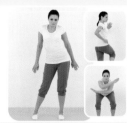 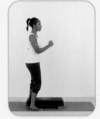 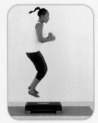

All 3 exercises, page 32
REPS: **16 of each**

PRESS-UPS

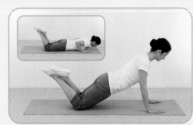 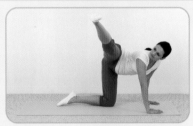

Tri press, page 65
REPS: **15**
INTENSITY: **Moderate**

STEP

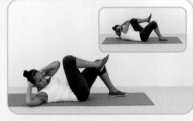

With jumps, page 37
REPS: **10**
INTENSITY: **Vigorous**

THIGH TONERS

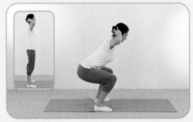

Circles, page 70
REPS: **10 on each leg**
INTENSITY: **Vigorous**

PLANK

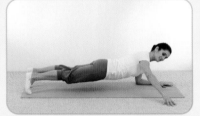

Touch line, page 42
TIME: **30 seconds while moving arms**
INTENSITY: **Vigorous**

SQUATS

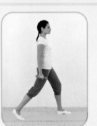

Prisoner squat, page 73
REPS: **10**
INTENSITY: **Moderate**

CURLS

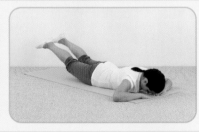

Diagonal curl, page 49
REPS: **15 on each alternating leg**
INTENSITY: **Moderate**

LUNGES

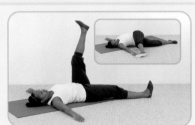

Forward step lunge, page 77
REPS: **10 on each leg**
INTENSITY: **Moderate**

HYPEREXTENSION

Leg fly, page 55
REPS: **8**
INTENSITY: **Moderate**

BODY STRETCH

Raised leg stretch, page 80
REPS/TIME: **1 on each side (hold for 10 seconds)**
INTENSITY: **Light**

ROLL DOWNS

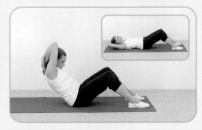

Necklace roll down, page 61
REPS: **3–4**
INTENSITY: **Moderate**

COOL DOWNS

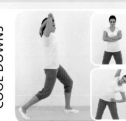

All 3 exercises, page 82
REPS/TIME: **1–2 of each (hold for 10–15 seconds with a feeling of mild tension)**

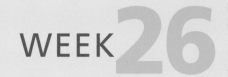
GOAL for this week... Check and recheck your posture – aim to lift and lengthen your spine

WARM UPS

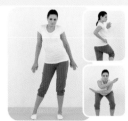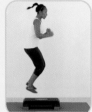

All 3 exercises, page 32
REPS: **16 of each**

STEP

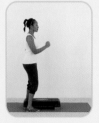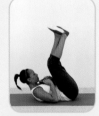

With jumps, page 37
REPS: **10**
INTENSITY: **Vigorous**

PLANK

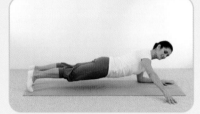

Touch line, page 42
TIME: **30 seconds while moving arms**
INTENSITY: **Vigorous**

CURLS

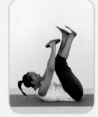

Weight lift, page 49
REPS: **20**
INTENSITY: **Moderate**

HYPEREXTENSION

Leg fly, page 55
REPS: **8**
INTENSITY: **Moderate**

ROLL DOWNS

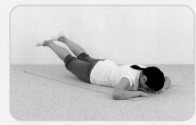

Necklace roll down, page 61
REPS: **3–4**
INTENSITY: **Moderate**

PRESS UPS

Tri press, page 65
REPS: **15**
INTENSITY: **Moderate**

THIGH TONERS

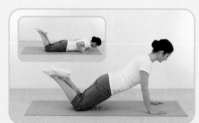

Circles, page 70
REPS: **10 on each leg**
INTENSITY: **Vigorous**

SQUATS

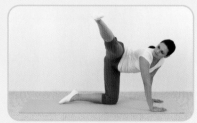

Prisoner squat, page 73
REPS: **10**
INTENSITY: **Moderts**

LUNGES

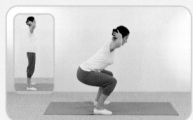

Forward step lunge, page 77
REPS: **10 on each leg**
INTENSITY: **Moderate**

BODY STRETCH

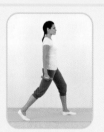

Raised leg stretch, page 80
REPS/TIME: **1 on each side (hold for 10 seconds)**
INTENSITY: **Light**

COOL DOWNS

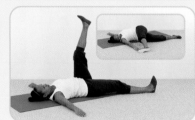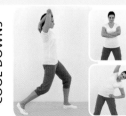

All 3 exercises, page 82
REPS/TIME: **1–2 of each (hold for 10–15 seconds with a feeling of mild tension)**

WARM UPS

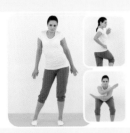

All 3 exercises, page 32
REPS: **16 of each**

PRESS UPS

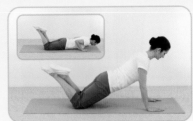

Tri press, page 65
REPS: **15**
INTENSITY: **Moderate**

STEP

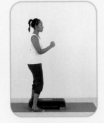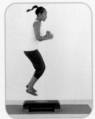

With jumps, page 37
REPS: **10**
INTENSITY: **Vigorous**

THIGH TONERS

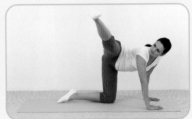

Circles, page 70
REPS: **10 on each leg**
INTENSITY: **Vigorous**

PLANK

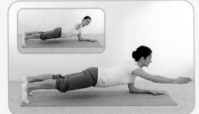

Semaphore, page 43
TIME: **30 seconds while moving arms**
INTENSITY: **Vigorous**

SQUATS

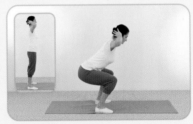

Prisoner squat, page 73
REPS: **10**
INTENSITY: **Moderate**

CURLS

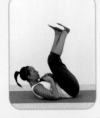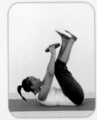

Weight lift, page 49
REPS: **20**
INTENSITY: **Moderate**

LUNGES

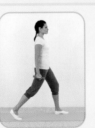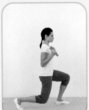

Forward step lunge, page 77
REPS: **10 on each leg**
INTENSITY: **Moderate**

HYPEREXTENSION

Leg fly, page 55
REPS: **8**
INTENSITY: **Moderate**

BODY STRETCH

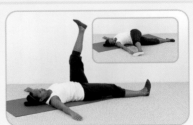

Raised leg stretch, page 80
REPS/TIME: **1 on each side (hold for 10 seconds)**
INTENSITY: **Light**

ROLL DOWNS

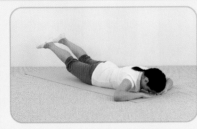

Necklace roll down, page 61
REPS: **3–4**
INTENSITY: **Moderate**

COOL DOWNS

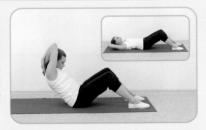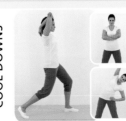

All 3 exercises, page 82
REPS/TIME: **1–2 of each (hold for 10–15 seconds with a feeling of mild tension)**

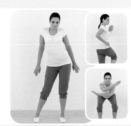

WARM UPS
All 3 exercises, page 32
REPS: **16 of each**

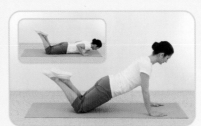
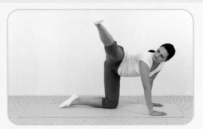

PRESS UPS
Tri press, page 65
REPS: **15**
INTENSITY: **Moderate**

STEP
Quick time, page 38
REPS: **10**
INTENSITY: **Vigorous**

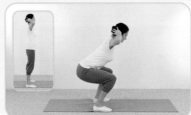

THIGH TONERS
Circles, page 70
REPS: **10 on each leg**
INTENSITY: **Vigorous**

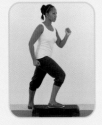

PLANK
Semaphore, page 43
TIME: **30 seconds while moving arms**
INTENSITY: **Vigorous**

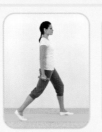

SQUATS
Prisoner squat, page 73
REPS: **10**
INTENSITY: **Moderate**

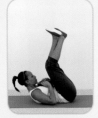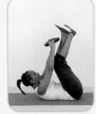

CURLS
Weight lift, page 49
REPS: **20**
INTENSITY: **Moderate**

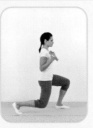

LUNGES
Forward step lunge, page 77
REPS: **10 on each leg**
INTENSITY: **Moderate**

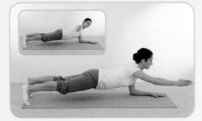

HYPEREXTENSION
Leg fly, page 55
REPS: **8**
INTENSITY: **Moderate**

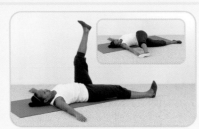

BODY STRETCH
Raised leg stretch, page 80
REPS/TIME: **1 on each side (hold for 10 seconds)**
INTENSITY: **Light**

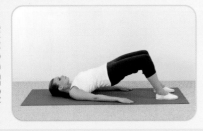

ROLL DOWNS
Hip arch, page 61
REPS: **6–8 slow roll ups**
INTENSITY: **Moderate**

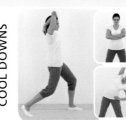

COOL DOWNS
All 3 exercises, page 82
REPS/TIME: **1–2 of each (hold for 10–15 seconds with a feeling of mild tension)**

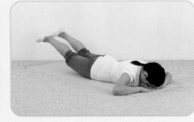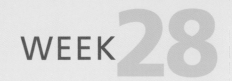

WARM UPS

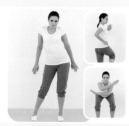

All 3 exercises, page 32
REPS: **16 of each**

PRESS UPS

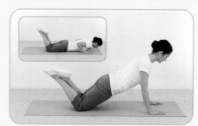

Tri press, page 65
REPS: **15**
INTENSITY: **Moderate**

STEP

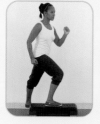

Quick time, page 38
REPS: **10**
INTENSITY: **Vigorous**

THIGH TONERS

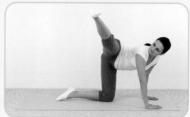

Circles, page 70
REPS: **10 on each leg**
INTENSITY: **Vigorous**

PLANK

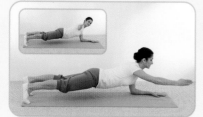

Semaphore, page 43
TIME: **30 seconds while moving arms**
INTENSITY: **Vigorous**

SQUATS

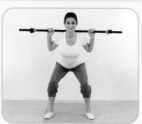

Barbell squat, page 74
REPS: **12 (hold for 1–2 seconds)**
INTENSITY: **Moderate**

CURLS

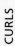
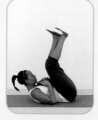
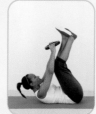

Weight lift, page 49
REPS: **20**
INTENSITY: **Moderate**

LUNGES

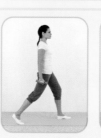

Forward step lunge, page 77
REPS: **10 on each leg**
INTENSITY: **Moderate**

HYPEREXTENSION

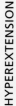

Leg fly, page 55
REPS: **8**
INTENSITY: **Moderate**

BODY STRETCH

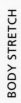
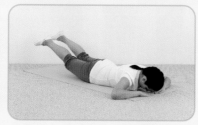

Sitting twist, page 81
REPS/TIME: **1 on each side (hold for 10 seconds)**
INTENSITY: **Light**

ROLL DOWNS

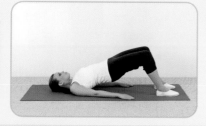

Hip arch, page 61
REPS: **6–8 slow roll ups**
INTENSITY: **Moderate**

COOL DOWNS

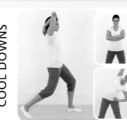

All 3 exercises, page 82
REPS/TIME: **1–2 of each (hold for 10–15 seconds with a feeling of mild tension)**

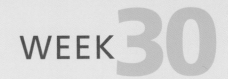

WARM UPS

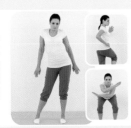

All 3 exercises, page 32
REPS: **16 of each**

PRESS UPS

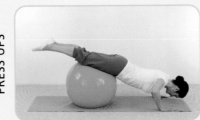

Ball press, page 66
REPS: **15**
INTENSITY: **Moderate**

STEP

Quick time, page 38
REPS: **10**
INTENSITY: **Vigorous**

THIGH TONERS

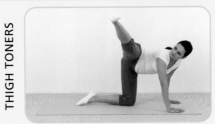

Circles, page 70
REPS: **10 on each leg**
INTENSITY: **Vigorous**

PLANK

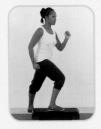

Semaphore, page 43
TIME: **30 seconds while moving arms**
INTENSITY: **Vigorous**

SQUATS

Barbell squat, page 74
REPS: **12 (hold for 1–2 seconds)**
INTENSITY: **Moderate**

CURLS

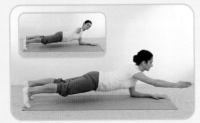

Lower ab tightener, page 50
REPS: **20 on each alternating leg**
INTENSITY: **Moderate**

LUNGES

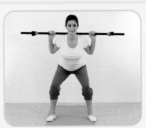

Forward step lunge, page 77
REPS: **10 on each leg**
INTENSITY: **Moderate**

HYPEREXTENSION

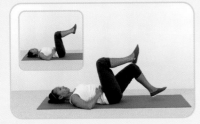

Leg fly, page 55
REPS: **8**
INTENSITY: **Moderate**

BODY STRETCH

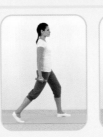

Sitting twist, page 81
REPS/TIME: **1 on each side (hold for 10 seconds)**
INTENSITY: **Light**

ROLL DOWNS

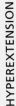
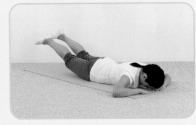

Hip arch, page 61
REPS: **6–8 slow roll ups**
INTENSITY: **Moderate**

COOL DOWNS

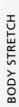
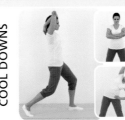
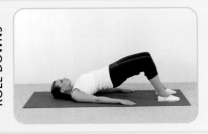
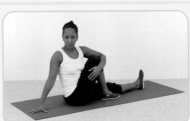

All 3 exercises, page 82
REPS/TIME: **1–2 of each (hold for 10–15 seconds with a feeling of mild tension)**

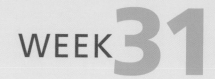
GOAL for this week... If you're feeling good, double the reps in the ab exercises

WARM UPS

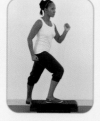

All 3 exercises, page 32
REPS: **16 of each**

PRESS UPS

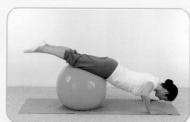

Ball press, page 66
REPS: **15**
INTENSITY: **Moderate**

STEP

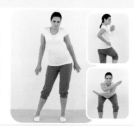

Quick time, page 38
REPS: **10**
INTENSITY: **Vigorous**

THIGH TONERS

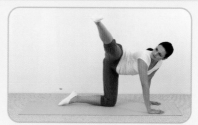

Circles, page 70
REPS: **10 on each leg**
INTENSITY: **Vigorous**

PLANK

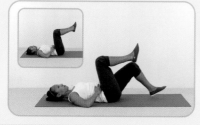

Semaphore, page 43
TIME: **30 seconds while moving arms**
INTENSITY: **Vigorous**

SQUATS

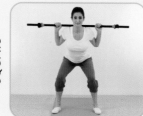

Barbell squat, page 74
REPS: **12 (hold for 1–2 seconds)**
INTENSITY: **Moderate**

CURLS

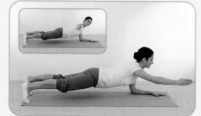

Lower ab tightener, page 50
REPS: **20 on each alternating leg**
INTENSITY: **Moderate**

LUNGES

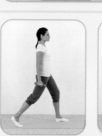

Forward step lunge, page 77
REPS: **10 on each leg**
INTENSITY: **Moderate**

HYPEREXTENSION

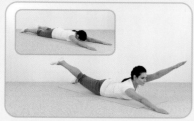 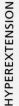

Dolphin lift, page 56
REPS: **1 on each side**
INTENSITY: **Moderate**

BODY STRETCH

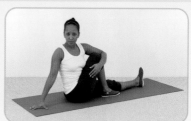

Sitting twist, page 81
REPS/TIME: **1 on each side (hold for 10 seconds)**
INTENSITY: **Light**

ROLL DOWNS

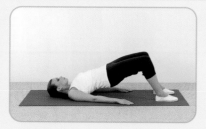

Hip arch, page 61
REPS: **6–8 slow roll ups**
INTENSITY: **Moderate**

COOL DOWNS

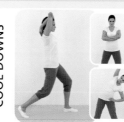

All 3 exercises, page 82
REPS/TIME: **1–2 of each (hold for 10–15 seconds with a feeling of mild tension)**

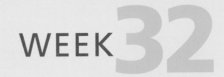
WARM UPS

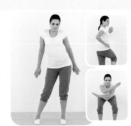

All 3 exercises, page 32
REPS: **16 of each**

PRESS UPS

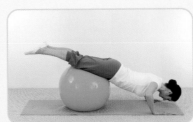

Ball press, page 66
REPS: **15**
INTENSITY: **Moderate**

STEP

Quick time, page 38
REPS: **10**
INTENSITY: **Vigorous**

THIG TONERS

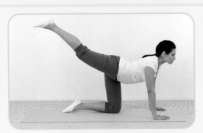

Leg swing, page 71
REPS: **15 on each leg**
INTENSITY: **Vigorous**

PLANK

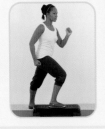

V-lifts, page 43
REPS: **10–15**
INTENSITY: **Vigorous**

SQUATS

Barbell squat, page 74
REPS: **12 (hold for 1–2 seconds)**
INTENSITY: **Moderate**

CURLS

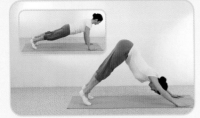

Lower ab tightener, page 50
REPS: **20 on each alternating leg**
INTENSITY: **Moderate**

LUNGES

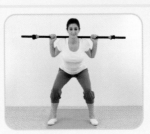

Forward step lunge, page 77
REPS: **10 on each leg**
INTENSITY: **Moderate**

HYPEREXTENSION

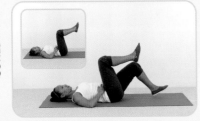

Dolphin lift, page 56
REPS: **1 on each side**
INTENSITY: **Moderate**

BODY STRETCH

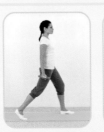

Sitting twist, page 81
REPS/TIME: **1 on each side (hold for 10 seconds)**
INTENSITY: **Light**

ROLL DOWNS

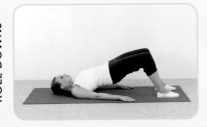

Hip arch, page 61
REPS: **6–8 slow roll ups**
INTENSITY: **Moderate**

COOL DOWNS

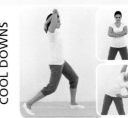

All 3 exercises, page 82
REPS/TIME: **1–2 of each (hold for 10–15 seconds with a feeling of mild tension)**

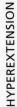

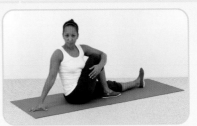
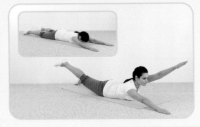

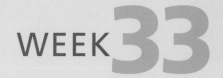

GOAL for this week... Sing while you work out to increase the cardiovascular challenge

WARM UPS

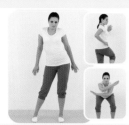 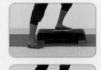

All 3 exercises, page 32
REPS: **16 of each**

PRESS UPS

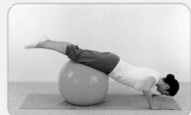

Ball press, page 66
REPS: **15**
INTENSITY: **Moderate**

STEP

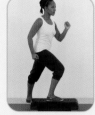

Quick time, page 38
REPS: **10**
INTENSITY: **Vigorous**

THIGH TONERS

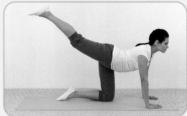

Leg swing, page 71
REPS: **15 on each leg**
INTENSITY: **Vigorous**

PLANK

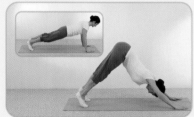

V-lifts, page 43
REPS: **10–15**
INTENSITY: **Vigorous**

SQUATS

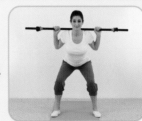

Barbell squat, page 74
REPS: **12 (hold for 1–2 seconds)**
INTENSITY: **Moderate**

CURLS

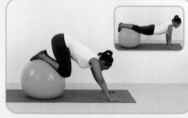

Ball ab buster, page 51
REPS: **10**
INTENSITY: **Vigorous**

LUNGES

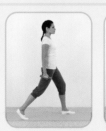 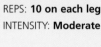

Forward step lunge, page 77
REPS: **10 on each leg**
INTENSITY: **Moderate**

HYPEREXTENSION

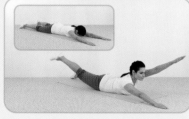 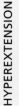

Dolphin lift, page 56
REPS: **1 on each side**
INTENSITY: **Moderate**

BODY STRETCH

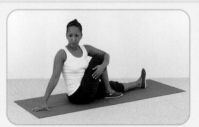

Sitting twist, page 81
REPS/TIME: **1 on each side (hold for 10 seconds)**
INTENSITY: **Light**

ROLL DOWNS

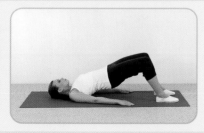

Hip arch, page 61
REPS: **6–8 slow roll ups**
INTENSITY: **Moderate**

COOL DOWNS

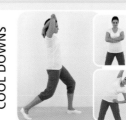

All 3 exercises, page 82
REPS/TIME: **1–2 of each (hold for 10–15 seconds with a feeling of mild tension)**

GOAL for this week... Concentrate on making all your swing movements really smooth

WEEK **34**

WARM UPS

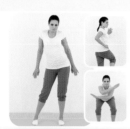

All 3 exercises, page 32
REPS: **16 of each**

PRESS UPS

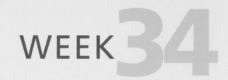

Full press up, page 66
REPS: **5, building up to 25**
INTENSITY: **Vigorous**

STEP

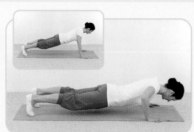

Quick time, page 38
REPS: **10**
INTENSITY: **Vigorous**

THIGH TONERS

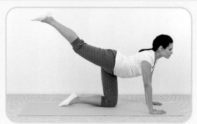

Leg swing, page 71
REPS: **15 on each leg**
INTENSITY: **Vigorous**

PLANK

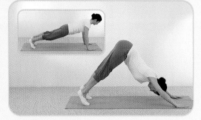

V-lifts, page 43
REPS: **10–15**
INTENSITY: **Vigorous**

SQUATS

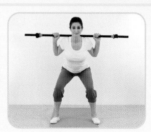

Barbell squat, page 74
REPS: **12 (hold for 1–2 seconds)**
INTENSITY: **Moderate**

CURLS

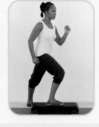

Half V-sit, page 51
REPS: **15 on each leg**
INTENSITY: **Vigorous**

LUNGES

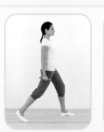

Forward step lunge, page 77
REPS: **10 on each leg**
INTENSITY: **Moderate**

HYPEREXTENSION

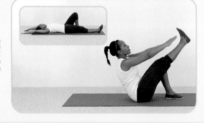

Dolphin lift, page 56
REPS: **1 on each side**
INTENSITY: **Moderate**

BODY STRETCH

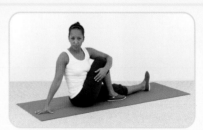

Sitting twist, page 81
REPS/TIME: **1 on each side (hold for 10 seconds)**
INTENSITY: **Light**

ROLL DOWNS

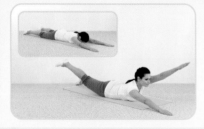

Hip arch & pulse, page 62
REPS: **5–15**
INTENSITY: **Moderate**

COOL DOWNS

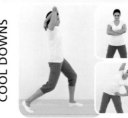

All 3 exercises, page 82
REPS/TIME: **1–2 of each (hold for 10–15 seconds with a feeling of mild tension)**

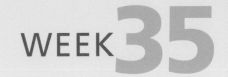

GOAL for this week... Pull up on the knees (lift the kneecaps) throughout all the exercises

WARM UPS

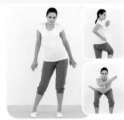

All 3 exercises, page 32
REPS: **16 of each**

STEP

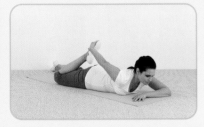

Quick time, page 38
REPS: **10**
INTENSITY: **Vigorous**

PLANK

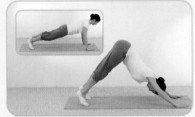

V-lifts, page 43
REPS: **10–15**
INTENSITY: **Vigorous**

CURLS

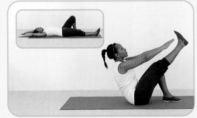

Half V-sit, page 51
REPS: **15 on each leg**
INTENSITY: **Vigorous**

HYPEREXTENSION

Quad hype, page 56
REPS: **4 on each side**
INTENSITY: **Moderate**

ROLL DOWNS

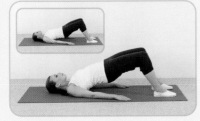

Hip arch & pulse, page 62
REPS: **5–15**
INTENSITY: **Moderate**

PRESS UPS

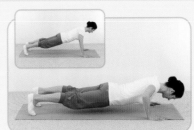
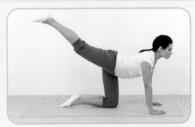

Full press up, page 66
REPS: **5, building up to 25**
INTENSITY: **Vigorous**

THIGH TONERS

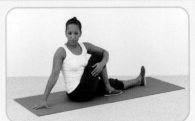

Leg swing, page 71
REPS: **15 on each leg**
INTENSITY: **Vigorous**

SQUATS

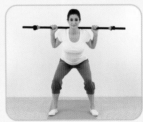

Barbell squat, page 74
REPS: **12 (hold for 1–2 seconds)**
INTENSITY: **Moderate**

LUNGES

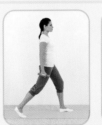

Forward step lunge, page 77
REPS: **10 on each leg**
INTENSITY: **Moderate**

BODY STRETCH

Sitting twist, page 81
REPS/TIME: **1 on each side (hold for 10 seconds)**
INTENSITY: **Light**

COOL DOWNS

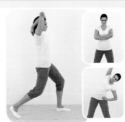

All 3 exercises, page 82
REPS/TIME: **1–2 of each (hold for 10–15 seconds with a feeling of mild tension)**

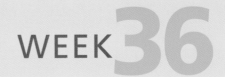
GOAL for this week...
Bend low to start so that you get a good high leap

WARM UPS

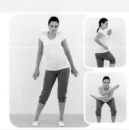

All 3 exercises, page 32
REPS: **16 of each**

STEP

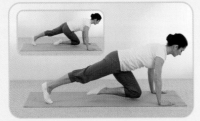

Quick time, page 38
REPS: **10**
INTENSITY: **Vigorous**

PLANK

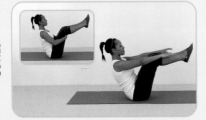

Mountain climbers,
page 44
REPS: **10–15,**
alternating legs
INTENSITY: **Vigorous**

CURLS

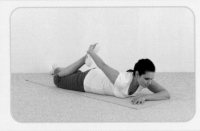

Full V-sit, page 52
TIME/REPS: **Lift & hold
for 5 seconds, repeat
5 times**
INTENSITY: **Vigorous**

HYPEREXTENSION

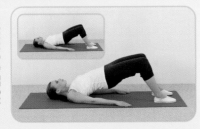
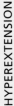

Quad hype, page 56
REPS: **4 on each side**
INTENSITY: **Moderate**

ROLL DOWNS

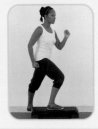

Hip arch & pulse,
page 62
REPS: **5–15**
INTENSITY: **Moderate**

PRESS UPS

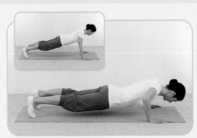

Full press up, page 66
REPS: **5, building up
to 25**
INTENSITY: **Vigorous**

THIGH TONERS

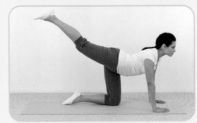

Leg swing, page 71
REPS: **15 on each leg**
INTENSITY: **Vigorous**

SQUATS

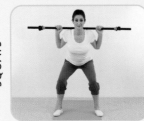

Barbell squat, page 74
REPS: **12 (hold for
1–2 seconds)**
INTENSITY: **Moderate**

LUNGES

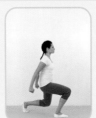

Leap lunge, page 77
REPS: **8 on each leg**
INTENSITY: **Vigorous**

BODY STRETCH

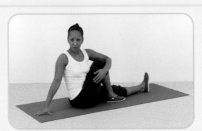

Sitting twist, page 81
REPS/TIME: **1 on each
side (hold for
10 seconds)**
INTENSITY: **Light**

COOL DOWNS

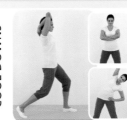

All 3 exercises, page 82
REPS/TIME: **1–2 of each (hold for
10–15 seconds with a feeling of
mild tension)**

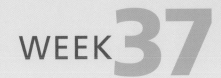

GOAL for this week...
If you're feeling good, add 5 to each rep count

WARM UPS

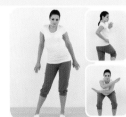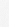

All 3 exercises, page 32
REPS: **16 of each**

STEP

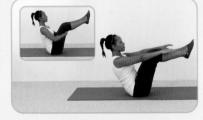

Quick time, page 38
REPS: **10**
INTENSITY: **Vigorous**

PLANK

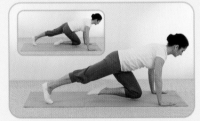

Mountain climbers, page 44
REPS: **10–15, alternating legs**
INTENSITY: **Vigorous**

CURLS

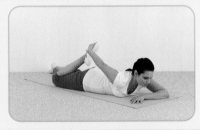

Full V-sit, page 52
TIME/REPS: **Lift & hold for 5 seconds, repeat 5 times**
INTENSITY: **Vigorous**

HYPEREXTENSION

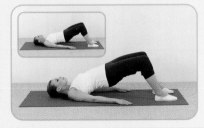

Quad hype, page 56
REPS: **4 on each side**
INTENSITY: **Moderate**

ROLL DOWNS

Hip arch & pulse, page 62
REPS: **5–15**
INTENSITY: **Moderate**

PRESS UPS

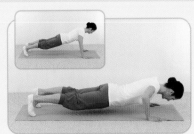

Full press up, page 66
REPS: **5, building up to 25**
INTENSITY: **Vigorous**

THIGH TONERS

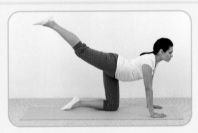

Leg swing, page 71
REPS: **15 on each leg**
INTENSITY: **Vigorous**

SQUATS

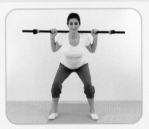

Barbell squat, page 74
REPS: **12 (hold for 1–2 seconds)**
INTENSITY: **Moderate**

LUNGES

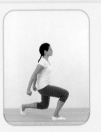

Leap lunge, page 77
REPS: **8 on each leg**
INTENSITY: **Vigorous**

BODY STRETCH

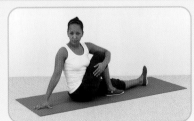

Sitting twist, page 81
REPS/TIME: **1 on each side (hold for 10 seconds)**
INTENSITY: **Light**

COOL DOWNS

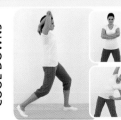

All 3 exercises, page 82
REPS/TIME: **1–2 of each (hold for 10–15 seconds with a feeling of mild tension)**

WARM UPS

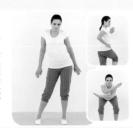 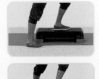 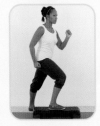

All 3 exercises, page 32
REPS: **16 of each**

PRESS UPS

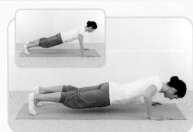 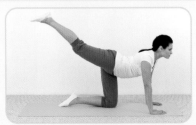

Full press up, page 66
REPS: **5, building up
to 25**
INTENSITY: **Vigorous**

STEP

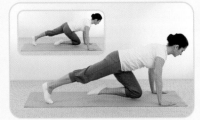

Quick time, page 38
REPS: **10**
INTENSITY: **Vigorous**

THIGH TONERS

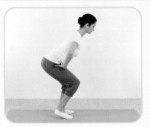

Leg swing, page 71
REPS: **15 on each leg**
INTENSITY: **Vigorous**

PLANK

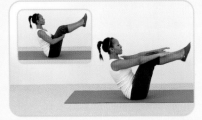

Mountain climbers,
page 44
REPS: **10–15,
alternating legs**
INTENSITY: **Vigorous**

SQUATS

One leg squat, page 74
REPS: **8 on each leg**
INTENSITY: **Vigorous**

CURLS

Full V-sit, page 52
TIME/REPS: **Lift & hold
for 5 seconds, repeat
5 times**
INTENSITY: **Vigorous**

LUNGES

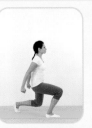 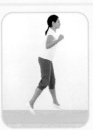

Leap lunge, page 77
REPS: **8 on each leg**
INTENSITY: **Vigorous**

HYPEREXTENSION

Quad hype, page 56
REPS: **4 on each side**
INTENSITY: **Moderate**

BODY STRETCH

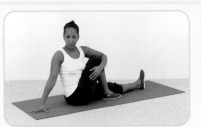

Sitting twist, page 81
REPS/TIME: **1 on each
side (hold for
10 seconds)**
INTENSITY: **Light**

ROLL DOWNS

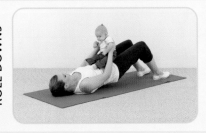 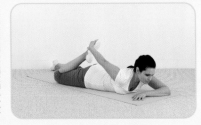

Baby hill top,
page 62
REPS: **10–12**
INTENSITY: **Moderate**

COOL DOWNS

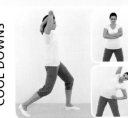

All 3 exercises, page 82
REPS/TIME: **1–2 of each (hold for
10–15 seconds with a feeling of
mild tension)**

GOAL for this week...
If you can, aim to add another 2 reps to each exercise

WARM UPS

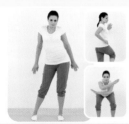

All 3 exercises, page 32
REPS: **16 of each**

PRESS UPS

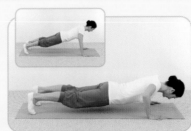

Full press up, page 66
REPS: **5, building up to 25**
INTENSITY: **Vigorous**

STEP

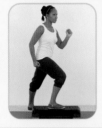

Quick time, page 38
REPS: **10**
INTENSITY: **Vigorous**

THIGH TONERS

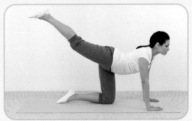

Leg swing, page 71
REPS: **15 on each leg**
INTENSITY: **Vigorous**

PLANK

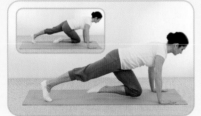

Mountain climbers, page 44
REPS: **10–15, alternating legs**
INTENSITY: **Vigorous**

SQUATS

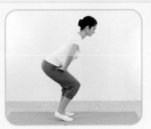

One leg squat, page 74
REPS: **8 on each leg**
INTENSITY: **Vigorous**

CURLS

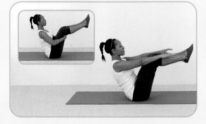

Full V-sit, page 52
TIME/REPS: **Lift & hold for 5 seconds, repeat 5 times**
INTENSITY: **Vigorous**

LUNGES

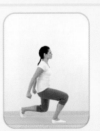

Leap lunge, page 77
REPS: **8 on each leg**
INTENSITY: **Vigorous**

HYPEREXTENSION

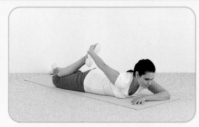

Quad hype, page 56
REPS: **4 on each side**
INTENSITY: **Moderate**

BODY STRETCH

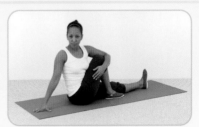

Sitting twist, page 81
REPS/TIME: **1 on each side (hold for 10 seconds)**
INTENSITY: **Light**

ROLL DOWNS

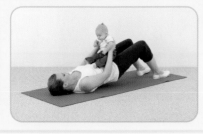

Baby hilltop, page 62
REPS: **10–12**
INTENSITY: **Moderate**

COOL DOWNS

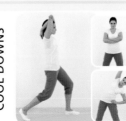

All 3 exercises, page 82
REPS/TIME: **1–2 of each (hold for 10–15 seconds with a feeling of mild tension)**

GOAL for this week... Concentrate on working every rep smoothly and with good technique

WARM UPS

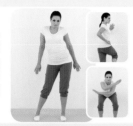

All 3 exercises, page 32
REPS: **16 of each**

STEP

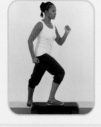

Quick time, page 38
REPS: **10**
INTENSITY: **Vigorous**

PLANK

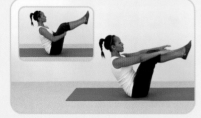

Spiderman, page 44
REPS: **10, alternating legs**
INTENSITY: **Vigorous**

CURLS

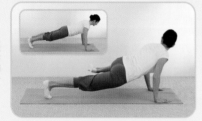

Full V-sit, page 52
TIME/REPS: **Lift & hold for 5 seconds, repeat 5 times**
INTENSITY: **Vigorous**

HYPEREXTENSION

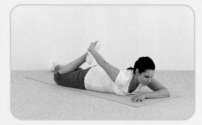

Quad hype, page 56
REPS: **4 on each side**
INTENSITY: **Moderate**

ROLL DOWNS

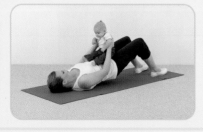

Baby hilltop, page 62
REPS: **10–12**
INTENSITY: **Moderate**

PRESS UPS

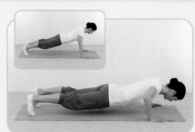

Full press up, page 66
REPS: **5, building up to 25**
INTENSITY: **Vigorous**

THIGH TONERS

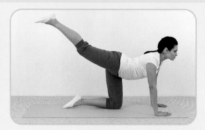

Leg swing, page 71
REPS: **15 on each leg**
INTENSITY: **Vigorous**

SQUATS

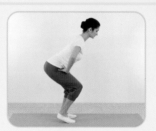

One leg squat, page 74
REPS: **8 on each leg**
INTENSITY: **Vigorous**

LUNGES

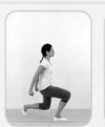

Leap lunge, page 77
REPS: **8 on each leg**
INTENSITY: **Vigorous**

BODY STRETCH

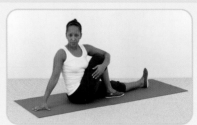

Sitting twist, page 81
REPS/TIME: **1 on each side (hold for 10 seconds)**
INTENSITY: **Light**

COOL DOWNS

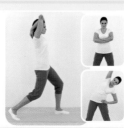

All 3 exercises, page 82
REPS/TIME: **1–2 of each (hold for 10–15 seconds with a feeling of mild tension)**

618.6   Gallagher-Mundy, Chrissie
GAL   Post pregnancy
         shape up

$19.95   9/14